FIRST PUBLISHED IN TH
STEP BY STEP REFLE
REVISED FOURTH EDI

CW00665070

COPYRIGHT 1990, 1998
© RENÉE TANNER

British Library - A CIP Catalogue record for this book is available from the British Library.

I.S.B.N. 0-9516203-5-5
Published in Great Britain by
Douglas Barry Publications,
21 Laud Street,
Croydon, Surrey.
CR0 1SU.

Film seperations by
Colourwise Ltd
Burgess Hill
Sussex

1

ABOUT THE AUTHOR

Renée Tanner is head of training for the Renbardou Group based at their head office in Croydon, Surrey. With almost 30 years of experience within the profession, she is a lecturer and author of international repute. Renée is also well respected for her numerous contributions to Radio, Television and Journals (publications for both the profession and for general public magazines).

ACKNOWLEDGEMENTS

I am indebted to many people who assisted me in the writing of this book.

Firstly I would like to thank my family, especially my daughter-in-law Samantha, for all the time, energy and constant encouragement given during the writing of the manuscript.

Also my many Clients, Friends, and Students both past and present who encouraged me to put my ideas down on paper and without whom this book might never have been written.

Finally I wish to place on record my thanks and appreciation for the help support and encouragement given to me by my late friend Anneke Van Der Mey.

CONTENTS

INTRODUCTION

While staying in Africa during 1973/4 I came into contact with a lady who was very interested in alternative therapies. Knowing my background in the Health and Beauty profession she lent me a book to read "Stories The Feet Can Tell", which had been written in 1938 by the famous American Reflexologist Eunice Ingham.

I was particularly fascinated by the book because as a child in Ireland, where folk medicine and folk-lore were part of life, I had met so many people who had the cure for so many ills. There were cures for "warts, the pains and chilblains" to name but a few and the bone setter was always on hand for the slipped disc or broken leg whether it be man or beast that was affected.

In my own case I had been told to massage my feet for chilblains and wear sheep's wool in my shoes.

For headaches we massaged our thumbs or around the base of the head (The Occipital) or around the eyes.

For worries such as school exams my late mother told me to massage my hands and wring them out. I still find myself following that same routine of hand massage these many years on. I realised on reading the Eunice Ingham Book that my hand massage of childhood bore a remarkable resemblance to the massage being described in Eunice Ingham's book.

On pointing out my interest to Edie who had given me the book, she invited me to learn the subject "first hand." Her knowledge had been gained from years of interest in the subject of health both through the natives of Africa and an American medical couple she had met in Zambia in the early sixties. I worked with and learned from Edie during the year that followed. When I left Africa in the summer of 1974 Edie gave me her proud possession of documented case studies. I placed them together with the many studies I had now collected for myself in an old brown attaché case to carry back with me to England rather than entrust them to transport with the risk of getting lost.

On the overland journey home to England while I ate my supper in a small outback hotel in the Province of Natal my car window was broken and the brown attaché case which had been carefully hidden under some blankets in the rear of our family estate was stolen, together with the blankets I had used to disguise them.

To my husband's delight however, all the camera equipment, which also lay beneath the blankets remained intact and untouched.

On my return to England my interest in the subject grew, as did my expansion of friends, though some were very sceptical at first.

In 1975 when Doreen Bailey gave me two treatments for sciatica, a condition that reared its ugly head after the birth of my second son in 1967, the results of the treatment served only to strengthen my belief and determination to succeed in spreading the knowledge and treatment.

Doreen and I spent some time on each of my two visits (2 complete days) discussing the treatment, its benefits and limitations; as well as ways in which we might educate the British public into recognizing the values of this ancient therapy. A further two days spent working with Doreen proved to be an invaluable experience for me.

During my many years gaining experience in Reflexology and having treated some thousands of people and personally trained numerous therapists (in latter years to pass the examinations of the International Examination Board, I.E.B. and for membership of the International Federation of Reflexologists, I.F.R.), I have been aware that there is still a need for a simple to follow guide on a no nonsense routine which will also help to dispel some of the mystery which surrounds this treatment.

Reflexology is a treatment that can be performed by most people; especially those who are prepared to study a basic course in anatomy and physiology and use their common sense with regard to orthodox medicine.

This book will be of help to the lay person who wishes to treat family and friends and also an asset to the Student or Qualified Therapist who wishes to work as a Professional.

HISTORY BEGINNINGS AND PROGRESS OF REFLEXOLOGY

Egypt, India, China, Russia, Japan, Native American Indians, Europe. All of these peoples have stories to tell about foot and hand treatments

America

With American Indians (Cherokee tribes) the tradition of treating the whole body by treating the feet in a specific way has been passed down through the generations and is still openly practised within the tribes.

Britain

Sir Henry Head published in 1893 his discoveries about the correspondence between spinal segments, skin sensitivity and internal organs. The bladder he wrote, can be exited into action by stimulating the soles of the feet. Charles Sherrington and Edgar Adrian explored the way the nervous system co-ordinates and dominates the body functions and activities. Sherrington established that the brain and its nerves co-ordinated and controlled body functions through transmission of impulses.

China

The ancient Chinese use many specific points on the feet to initiate healing. Chinese massage as in Indian massage pays particular attention to treating points on the feet. Ancient Chinese acupuncture treated many points on the feet.

Egypt

The Egyptians can trace their history of foot reflexology back to 2500BC. According to the illustrated papyrus from that time, the medical practitioner of the day can be seen treating their patients hands and feet.
A wall hieroglyphic in the tomb of the physician Ankhmahor is depicting a form of foot treatment being given.

Europe

In 1582 Dr Adamus and Dr Atatis published a book on zone therapy, through these writings we are aware of a form of reflex therapy being practised in the countries of Central Europe.

Greece and Italy

Greeks and Romans do not seem to have evidenced written records of specific foot treatments, though we are aware of a strong history of massage. A number of medical documents are believed to have been destroyed in the fires of Alexandria.

India

The peoples of India performed a form of pressure technique on the feet as part of their system of Ayurvedic medicine. These traditions live on through oral exchange and skills demonstration from generation to generation.

Russia and Germany

These peoples made huge contributions to general reflex actions between body parts and developed various applications for treatment. Reflex massage was developed the results of the treatment was then credited to the result of reflex actions. Dr Alfonse Cornelius is credited with the discovery that spending time treating a painful part contributed to the improvement of health and the elimination of pain.

USA

Medical Dr's William Fitzgerald and Edwin Bowers are generally acknowledged as the forefathers of modern reflexology. Influenced by Fitzgeralds trips abroad and by the Cherokee tribes of his native New England. Fitzgerald was head of the Ear Nose and Throat unit at St. Francis hospital Hartford, Connecticut. Fitzgerald as early as 1917 discovered that pressure on the hands and/or feet produced pain relief in distant parts of the body and the condition causing the pain was also relieved.

Bowen demonstrate how he could apply pressure to a point on the hand or foot to the area corresponding to the face and then stick a pin in the face without causing intolerable pain if indeed any pain.
Fitzgerald went on to confirm that the parts of the body which had such reflex relationships lay within longitudinal zones or channels, he traced ten of these zone lines through the body and called his therapy 'Zone Therapy'. Similar to Head, Fitzgerald found that working within a zonal area affected everything along that zone and published his findings in medical journals. Most of his medical colleagues either ridiculed or ignored his ideas. One colleague, Dr Jo Riley learned the technique from Fitzgerald and taught the technique to his wife Elizabeth and to a young employee massage therapist Eunice Ingham.

Riley and Ingham gradually lessened the emphasis on Zone Therapy spending more time on the ancient pressure point theory. Between them they developed a routine for treatment which Ingham perfected to her own liking. Elizabeth Riley practised a slightly different routine adding rotary pressure points and twists into her routine, however both women were still working on the ancient pressure points, just the method of deliverance of the treatment differed.

Elizabeth Riley remained working in her husbands practice developing her treatment, while Eunice took the therapy to the non medical public across the length and breath of the USA. In 1938 Eunice Ingham published two books 'Stories the Feet Can Tell' and 'Stories the Feet Have Told.'

Eunice often faced harassment from the medical profession. At the age of 80 years (1968) Eunice was charged and faced a possible court case in New York for practising medicine without a licence. The charges against this frail elderly lady were dropped before the final court action. It is generally believed that her advancing years had a bearing on the charges being dropped.

Eunice later retired completely from treating and teaching the public self help reflexology. She died in 1974. Ironically this is the year I added Reflexology to my school curriculum.

My own history in relation to reflexology began in 1973 and I felt confident to add this therapy to my school curriculum in 1974. I first studied the therapy in Africa where foot massage seemed to be just another natural therapy. My tutor Edith Holmes passed on the knowledge she had gained from her lifelong understanding of the African way of life and also from the knowledge and skill she had learned from American, Chinese, and Indian missionaries over her lifetime in Africa.

I do not teach the Ingham method of treatment though there are similarities like her I developed my own technique and routine, practised on my eleven thousand case studies.

My own theories are based on a sound knowledge and understanding of Anatomy and Physiology, supported by a life times experience investigating disorders and diseases which began in my childhood in my native Irish village. On my return from Africa I met and worked with Doreen Baily a former student of Eunice Ingham and the first person to teach the therapy to the British public which she began doing in the early seventies, having practised the therapy herself from 1966.

This text book Step By Step Reflexology (4th Edition) the first of its kind ever published is based on my routine and completely documents a full treatment in simple to understand language supported with line drawings. It is now published in a number of languages and sales worldwide have now surpassed my wildest dreams. I note that a number of books which have proceeded my own carry information and text in imitation of my own with no reference to its originality, this I do not challenge but live in the hope that those who read and practice this method will gain the desired results.

Having opened the first Beauty and Complementary Therapy Training Centre in the UK I gained a lot of experience in teaching which I later expanded into many countries worldwide.

The International Federation of Reflexologists has honoured me with Chairmanship for a number of years. I have had the joy to see this professional body grow into an outstanding organisation with high educational and skills requirements.

Today's progress sees the IFR with a Post Graduate training facility second to none; a research section, and ethics committee. Our strong overseas exchange committee maintains contact with our fellow therapists in many countries throughout the world. Our therapists telephone Support Line is kept very busy as is the Student and Public Help Line.

To conclude this chapter I would examine my own health which is, I am happy to report, excellent I attribute this incredible gift to the practice of reflexology.

My future wish is the continuation of post graduation training and integration of Reflexology into the NHS so all may benefit form this non-invasive therapy.

REFLEXOLOGY EXPLAINED

Reflexology is a specific pressure technique applied to the feet or hands where all the internal body structures and organs are mapped or mirrored in minature. It is a simple non-invasive treatment which helps the body to maintain a delicate balance between the nine systems.

Skeletal
Muscular
Vascular
Neurological
Respiratory
Digestive
Endocrine
Urinary
Reproductive
All these systems work together in harmony and unison to keep us in a state of good health.

No one knows exactly how Reflexology works, although many theories exist. Most Reflexologists subscribe to the theory that the body is divided into ten longitudinal zones (or energy pathways/zones). These zones are lines running the entire length of the body; five on each side of the median line (an imaginary line running from the crown of the head to between the feet-see diagram 'A'-page 15).

These zones extend into the feet which are also divided into ten zones, five on each foot. (see diagram 'D' - page 17). The foot zones are located with number one on the first toe (big toe) counting to number five on the little toe. These lines are repeated, running down the arm to the fingers. On the hands number one zone or channel runs to the thumb and number five to the little finger.

On each foot and hand are found areas known as reflex points corresponding to each gland and structure in the body.

The hands and feet have the same reflex zones and points, however from working experience there is no doubt that treatment of the feet gives better therapeutic results than does treatment of the hands. Whilst all therapists believe in the benefits of the treatment there are some who believe that because of the mobility of the hand the reflexes are not so clearly defined and also the hands are much smaller so specific reflex points are more difficult to locate. Yet another school of thought is that because the total body weight passes through the feet and as the feet are more protected from the elements the energy channels and reflex points are more sensitive to touch.

The reflex points of Reflexology differ from the neurological reflex points; they do not cross the spinal column and are invisible on dissection. Zones are not visible on X-ray.

It could therefore be said that in this instance reflex is taken to mean the reflection of the organs and structures of the body in miniature on the feet.

Energy chi or qi (pronounced chee) flows through each zone/channel. When the energy flow is blocked by congestion disorder and even disease can occur. When the therapist treats a reflex point the main aim is to enhance the energy flow encouraging the body to heal itself and the systems to work again in unison. Another benefit of the therapy is to break down tiny waste deposits (known as crystals) that can sometimes be found at reflex points (especially joints) and encourage their removal through the normal elimination process.

Besides the ten energy channels already mentioned three further lines should be taken into consideration. These are the imaginary lateral lines that traverse the foot or hand (See diagram 'B' - page 16). These lines help the Reflexologist to make a map of the foot or indeed the body. It is worth bearing in mind that the shape and size of feet differ in each individual. Therefore if treatment is always started by first visualising these three imaginary lines on the feet then it is easy to work out the reflexes that are above or below these lines.

1 The Diaphragm Line	Just below the ball of the foot.
2 The Waist Line.	In the centre of the arch. As a guide find the protrusion on outside of foot (base of 5th matatarsal)
3 The Pelvic Floor Line.	On the heel where thickness of the flesh changes to softness.

All organs and structures above the diaphragm on the body will have their reflex point above the diaphragm line on the foot and all organs below the diaphragm will have the reflex point in the corresponding area on the foot.

These three horizontal or transverse lines could logically be placed almost anywhere on the foot by a therapist with a very good working knowledge of anatomy and physiology. However the most commonly used three lines, which in turn form compartments for the organs of areas of the body, are the ones mentioned and are the ones which I personally use.

The alternative area commonly used is the shoulder girdle line but this is more difficult to find, especially for the novice.

Organs/structures on the right side of the body will be found in the right foot and those on the left side of the body found in the left foot.

Where two organs exist, for example two lungs, then they will be found one on each foot.

Likewise where an organ crosses the midline in the body it will then be found on both feet.

The reflex zone to an organ can be found occupying the same vertical body zone in the feet as the organ occupies in the body.

Important Note !
The Renée Tanner Reflexology Treatment Sequence described in this book is actually treating the whole body including all the reflex points. Further treatments of a specific reflex point is also included here as a backup concentrating on the actual point/area of the reflex which has proven to give the most satisfactory results without over stimulating a particular reflex. An example of this being the heart which is treated in its entirety in the general sequence routine of the chest, it is then backed up on the left foot only, though in reality the heart actually crosses the median line in the body. Hence in Reflexology a small portion is being represented on the right foot Z1 above the diaphragm line, but to concentrate on this area by returning to treat the area again/specifically would cause a healing crisis in some people and may over stimulate the heart reflex in others.

THE WORKING THERAPIST

All Reflexologists whether working for family and friends or as professional therapists, need to have a basic knowledge of anatomy and physiology as well as a knowledge of disorders and diseases. The professional therapist needs to have a very good working knowledge of these subjects and should study to the accepted standard. Therapists with membership of the International Federation of Reflexologists will have undertaken a course of study in Anatomy & Physiology equivalent to 'A' level standard and in excess of that required for nursing.

The I.F.R. require that students undertake a considerable number of hours of case study work before embarking on a career as a therapist. I would always advise that if you are treating others in a professional capacity you undertake a full course of training in that subject to a qualifying standard and never offer any treatment or part of any treatment beyond that in which you hold a qualification.

It is true to say that a qualified therapist will not mix his/her therapies in any one session. No more than a client/patient would have an osteopathic treatment and a chiropractic treatment on the same day he or she should not be given any other two therapies on the same day, however a qualified Reflexologists who is also a qualified aromatherapist might prescribe aromatherapy oils for home care i.e. bath oils. I am not however, suggesting that a reflexology treatment and an aromatherapy treatment should be given at the same time. I believe to do so would be demonstrating a lack of full understanding of Reflexology and I am supported in this view by many eminent reflexologists of today.

Do bear in mid that reflexology is not a "cure all" to the exclusion of other therapies and to insist on it being so indicates a lack of ability to evaluate the relative worth of different possibilities.

SOME BENEFITS OF REFLEXOLOGY

Reduces feelings of stress

Calms and soothes

Gives the recipient a feeling of wellbeing

Relaxes mind and body

Encourages elimination

Improves circulation

Assists the body in maintaining a balanced state

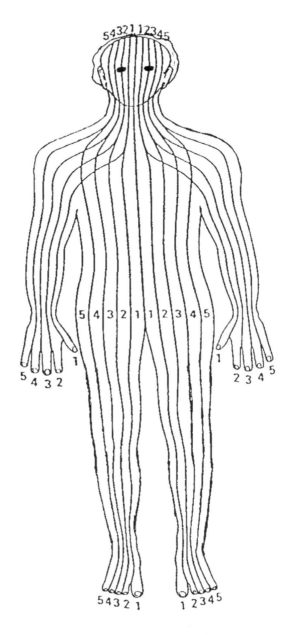

DIAGRAM A

15

TRANSVERSE LINES

RIGHT FOOT   LEFT FOOT

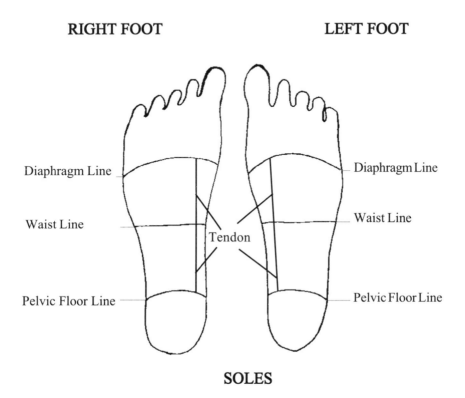

Diaphragm Line —   — Diaphragm Line

Waist Line —   — Waist Line

                    Tendon

Pelvic Floor Line —   — Pelvic Floor Line

SOLES

DIAGRAM 'B'

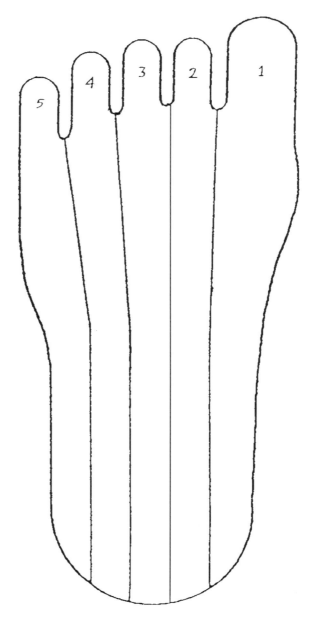

ZONES OF THE FOOT

DIAGRAM 'D'

MIRROR OF THE BODY

THE STRUCTURE OF THE FOOT

7	Tarsals	**NOTE.**
5	Metatarsals	Only 2 Phalanges in
14	Phalanges	the big toe.

Besides these 26 bones the foot also contains approximately :

    20   Muscles
    50   Ligaments
    500   Blood vessels
          Thousands of nerve endings

The bones of the foot are so arranged as to produce three distinct arches :

The Medial Longitudinal Arch.
This is the highest of the arches and is formed by the :
    Talus
    Calcaneus
    Navicular
    Three Cuneiform bones
    Metatarsals 1,2,3.

Only the Calcaneus and the distal end of the Metatarsals should touch the ground.

The Lateral Longitudinal Arch
This is much less marked than the Medial Arch and is composed of the :
    Calcaneus
    Cuboid and
    Metatarsals 4,5.

The Transverse Arch
This arch is formed by the :
    Navicular
    Three Cuneiforms
    Cuboid
    Five Metatarsals

The Arches are not fixed and they give as the weight of the body is transmitted to the ground. When the weight is removed they return to their original state.

The bones comprising the arches are held in position by ligaments and tendons. When these ligaments and tendons are weakened the height of the Medial Longitudinal Arch may decrease or 'fall' causing Flat Foot.

THE STRUCTURE OF THE FOOT

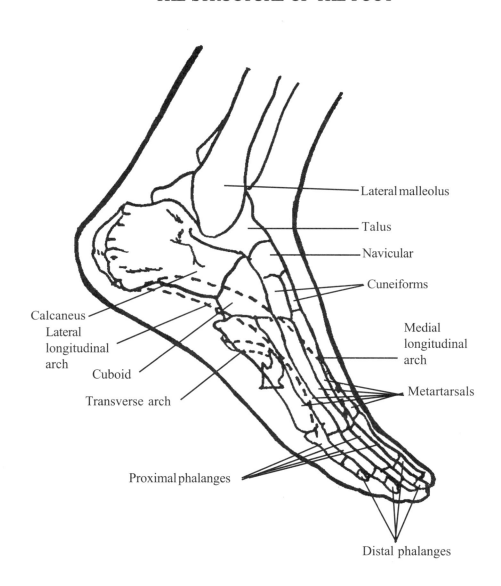

Lateral malleolus

Talus

Navicular

Cuneiforms

Calcaneus

Lateral longitudinal arch

Cuboid

Transverse arch

Medial longitudinal arch

Metartarsals

Proximal phalanges

Distal phalanges

**WEIGHT BEARING
BONES OF THE FOOT
OUTLINED BY
TRIANGLE**

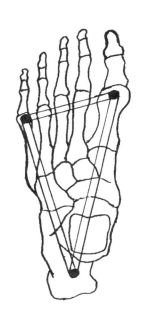

**CUSHIONED WEIGHT
BEARING AREA OF THE
FOOT**

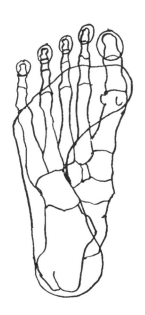

MUSCLES OF THE FIRST LAYER ON THE SOLE

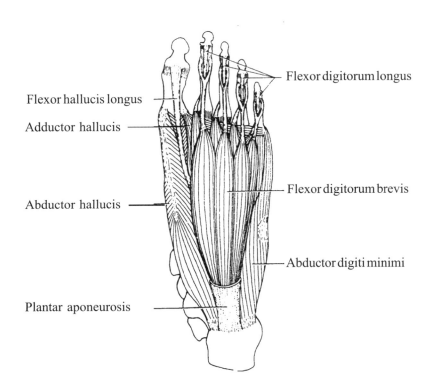

Flexor digitorum longus

Flexor hallucis longus

Adductor hallucis

Flexor digitorum brevis

Abductor hallucis

Abductor digiti minimi

Plantar aponeurosis

REFERRAL ZONES

Referral zones are an important part of treatment, particularly when treating oneself or dealing with cases of injury or infection; when the normal area cannot be treated.

For Example problems arising in :

Fingers Treat Toes

Hands Treat Foot

Wrist Treat Ankle

Forearm Treat Calf

Elbow Treat Knee

Upper Arm Treat Thigh

Shoulder Treat Hip

Naturally these treatments can be performed in reverse order. In the case of a Knee injury one could treat the Elbow; and so on.

When you know the Longitudinal Zones then the next step is to trace the zone in which that part of the body lies that is causing the problem. A general massage of the Referral Zone should bring relief to the area of the body that is out of tune (see diagram 'C' - page24).

It is worth bearing in mind that **self-treatment**, while being helpful, will never be as beneficial as a treatment given by another; as it is impossible to achieve the same degree of relaxation and equally as difficult to perceive one's own bodily reactions.

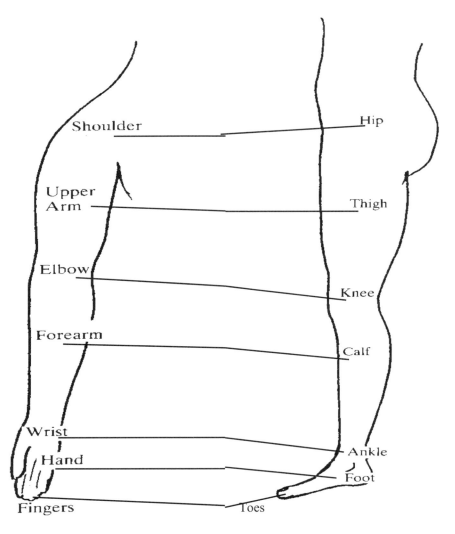

Shoulder

Hip

Upper
Arm

Thigh

Elbow

Knee

Forearm

Calf

Wrist

Ankle

Hand

Foot

Fingers

Toes

REFERRAL ZONES

DIAGRAM 'C '

WHAT DOES SENSITIVITY INDICATE ?

Sensitivity indicates congestion/energy blockage, the more sensitive the area is the more congested it is likely to be. Sensitivity and reactions will vary from person to person. I am sometimes asked, 'Will all clients have sensitivity on most visits?' No, especially on the first or second visit, nothing much is felt in some people. This may mean an energy blockage in the feet which needs to be freed before the full benefits of Reflexology can be appreciated or it could be due to a number of factors such as :

a.   How a person perceives hurt/pain or sensitivity;

b.   If there is a strong analgesic (pain killing) drug being taken;

c.   The recipient may not be prepared to accept treatment at the moment

d.   Reflexology not being a cure all may not be suitable for this particular person. However, in these cases, at least three treatments should be given before deciding on the suitability or likely effectiveness of Reflexology.

WHAT ARE THE CRYSTALS (GRITTY BITS) ?

Uric Acid and excess Calcium are two of the waste products that build up in the body when the metabolism is not working according to plan. These deposits can be felt on the feet (usually near joints) as grains of sugar or sand. The little clumps can be broken down by the Reflexology technique. The broken down deposits are then carried by the blood and lymph flow to be eliminated by the body. Crystals are on the whole found on or near joints.

WHEN TREATMENTS MUST NOT BE PERFORMED OR WHEN MEDICAL ADVICE SHOULD BE SOUGHT

This list of contra indications and precautions is meant to be a guide and is in no way to be taken as full and complete. The responsibility for the client rests with the therapist using his/her common sense at all times.

For any condition currently being treated by a medically qualified person without first obtaining that person's consent.

Immediately prior to surgery as treatment might cause a healing crisis.

Directly after surgery due to the risk of thrombosis. (12 to 24 hours should elapse)

Pregnancy. Where there is any element of risk and never without medical consent. Great care should be taken and all movements should be light. I personally do not recommend that Reflexology treatment be given in the first 12/14 weeks of pregnancy by anyone with less than three years of proven clinical experience in this therapy. The benefits of Reflexology in labour are mentioned on page 26. During pregnancy **specific** treatment of the hypothalamus, pituitary, ovaries, uterus and liver should be omitted but obviously these areas will be treated in the general routine (stroking the reflex of uterus and ovaries)

In cases of contagious/acute infections, condition/disease

Undiagnosed pain especially acute - Medical advice needed.

Thrombosis, Phlebitis - Medical advice needed.

Directly over an area of varicose veins, bruises, cuts, painful areas or recent scars.

After a heavy meal allow a couple of hours before treating otherwise mild abdominal pain/discomfort might be experienced.

On an empty stomach. Offer a glass of fruit juice and a biscuit.(mild pain otherwise).

On a person under the influence of the abuse of Alcohol or Drugs. (see 'Teacher Tell Me Why' on page 190 No.24)

During client/patient menstruation if it is normally very heavy.

For any rare or unusual condition without prior medical consent.

Internal bleeding

Gangrene of legs/feet

AIDS (unless the therapist has full knowledge of the condition)

Advice on AIDS. Light pressure, plenty of effleurage/holds/stroking. Know and understand the condition before attempting to treat (experience in counselling is helpful). I do not wear gloves. Reflexology is about human contact and touch; common sense is necessary as is the observance of all the hygiene rules and regulations. If in doubt contact a GP/patient support group or the International Federation of Reflexologists.

Student therapists must not treat AIDS patients without first taking advice from a senior tutor.

Remember! It is not within the skill of a Reflexologist to make a medical diagnosis. That is the prerogative of the medically qualified or others recognised to do so.

WHEN TO EXERCISE CAUTION

Epileptics. Client might have a fit. Can you cope? Can the epileptic cope? What are the risks if the client/patient does have a seizure?

When working on a diabetic use less pressure than normal and in severe cases, work for only about twenty to twenty five minutes with reflexology. Care should be taken in the pancreas area (treated with stomach). Beware of hypoglycaemia/ hyperglycaemia.

Do not treat diabetics with pressure circles on sensitive points but hold and release once.

Diabetics have a slow healing rate; heavy pressure might cause bruising.

The skin is easily broken or torn. Should this happen then the person might get a varicose ulcer.

It is possible to release too many toxins for the system to cope with and this can make the diabetic feel ill (strong healing crisis).

Under normal circumstances when the client is very sensitive to touch or has a lot of waste deposits collected in the joints good judgement is required with duration of treatment and pressures, otherwise the reactions from the client will be similar to that of the diabetic client. (Strong healing reaction - a feeling of being unwell).

In order to overcome this it is advisable to treat the client for a shorter period of time, increasing the pressure circles from one or two to begin with to the normal number as the course progresses. This should give the body a chance to disperse the toxins and encourage natural healing.

Pregnancy has been mentioned as a possible contra indication. It can however be a beneficial treatment especially during labour and immediately after delivery, providing there are no medical complications, the therapist is fully qualified and both patient and medical consent has been granted to allow the treatment to be performed. Treatment during pregnancy should only be carried out by an experienced therapist.

Unstable blood pressure. Regular monitoring by a doctor is advised.

Manic depression/paranoia psychosis. Therapist should have professional counselling skills and experience in this field.

On clients with decalcification of bone, osteoporosis or fractures. Great care must be taken. Avoid direct contact with the injury and work lightly.

On a person taking strong medication (advise client to get medical advice) pressure must be very light. Intervals between treatments might need to be longer. Caution is necessary to avoid the possibility of expelling important medication.

All practitioners of Reflexology should be aware not only of its benefits but also of its limitations.

It is of the utmost importance to exercise caution when dealing with the health of others.

Be prepared to refer people to their doctor or other practitioners when necessary.

Never make a medical diagnosis.

Never make false claims for the treatment.

And above all, never give false hope.

When treating children light pressures should be used (remember legal and ethical requirements).

Take extra care when dealing with Children, the Elderly, the Terminally Ill, Diabetics, Unusual Conditions, Acute Conditions (know and do not treat the notifiable diseases without special medical consent).

SOME DO'S AND DO NOT'S OF REFLEXOLOGY

THE DO NOT'S

Work on tendons or bone (with heavy pressure)

Work on infected areas.

Work on broken skin.

Work over surface veins with pressure.

Work over recent scar tissue.

Increase greatly the depth of pressure when you feel sensitivity or get a crystal reaction.

Hurt client to extent of causing deep pain or discomfort.

Diagnose disorder or a disease.

Give false hope.

Make false claims.

Have a flustered, rushed or hurried approach to your work.

Discuss one client with another.

Abuse your professional position.

Set up and work as a professional Reflexologist unless you have the necessary training, hold the qualification of a recognised examinations authority, and belong to a professional organisation.

SOME DO'S AND DO NOT'S OF REFLEXOLOGY

THE DO'S

Take care of your client/patient.

Give each and every client/patient your undivided attention.

Explain the therapy.

Be honest as far as possible.

Advise on code of confidentiality.

Have a warm, clean and relaxed atmosphere to work in.

Have a soothing, calm, quiet voice.

Explain clearly to the client what you would like them to do. For example remove shoes, socks, tights, lie down, bend leg.

Give a helping hand to the less able in removing shoes and clothing.

Try to accommodate clients/patients who might have a strict timetable to adhere to. Parking meters, public transport or dental appointments do not wait.

Complete consultation card prior to treatment and therapy record card on completion of treatment (while client/patient is getting ready to leave, or immediately after their departure).

Respect your client's shyness.

Advise client to drink as much water as possible after the treatment.

KNOW YOUR RESPONSIBILITIES

If you take it upon yourself to tell your client/patient the precise organs/glands you are working on, then you should be prepared to take the consequences of your action. If the therapist does choose to give this information he/she should aim to support the reasoning by relating to the information given by the client during the consultation. i.e. a reaction found on the ear reflex may correspond to a recent cold.

Many clients/patients who seem calm, logical and sensible while in your company can be caused great anxiety when alone, thinking about your treatment and comments. Few people fully understand the principles of Reflexology and imagination is a powerful tool. The therapist should always be professional and ethical in his/her approach to work, especially in answering client's questions with regard to areas or organs being worked on.

Should a professional Reflexologist feel that the client/patient being treated would benefit by seeking medical advice, or that he/she should be referred to a therapist with different or more appropriate skills, then the professional Reflexologist is both morally and ethically bound to give this advice to his/her client/patient.

ABNORMALITIES OF THE FEET THAT AFFECT OTHER REFLEX ZONES

1. Infected toe nails normally indicate that the Reflex Zones to the head area have been affected. Sugar, alcohol or cigarette use might be high. Migraine could even be a problem.

2. Hammer Toes and similar deformities suggest the Head and Face Zones are or have been affected.

3. Flat feet would indicate the Reflex Zones to the Spinal Column are affected. There may also be some digestive problems such as constipation.

4. Congestion in the ankle area would indicate affected Reflex Zones in the Pelvis or Hip Joint.

5. Bunions/Hallux Vulgus. suggests possible congestion in the Reflex Zones of the Cervical and Thoracic Spine, the Thyroid and the Pancreas

6. Corns showing anywhere on the feet (whatever the initial cause) indicates that the Reflex Zone for that area might be affected. If the corn presents itself in the shoulder reflex point or similar area this would naturally tell us that there might well be a problem in the shoulder area but could also suggest congestion/energy blockage in the entire zone.

7. Athletes Foot (Tinea Pedis). Observe carefully. The spread of the infection may cover more than one zone. When there is infection present or there is a change of colour or texture radiating from that area it usually indicates an energy blockage in the affected zone. If athletes foot is present or if there is any doubt work on the client's/patient's hands but do examine the feet first.

8.   I believe that any change in the skeletal, muscular or tissue structure of the foot could, like Athletes Foot, suggest an energy blockage in the corresponding area of the body. Therefore even if the client does not complain of problems within an area where we get visible signs of such, it is still worthwhile to work on those areas even if the skin is thick. Eventually we should get results. Alternatively instead of working on areas of hard skin work on the corresponding area on the hand after you have completed the foot routine. (Never break from the foot routine to treat the hand).

TIMING YOUR TREATMENTS

The professional therapist is not treating people only because he or she believes in what they are doing but also in order to earn their living. Therefore it is of great importance to get oneself well organised at the beginning of the day.

I always make a one and a half hour appointment for a client/patient on their first visit. This allows me to give a consultation and deal with any unexpected eventuality that might arise on the first day. It is extremely difficult to be precise in timing treatments thereafter; so for this reason it is best to allow one hour for every client. I work on the premise of ten minutes for preparation; five at the beginning and end of each treatment.

Some clients/patients can take, and indeed some need, a full treatment of forty to forty-five minutes. Yet there is the client who is so sensitive that five or ten minutes is all they can endure without a break, especially on a first or second visit.

Always allow the client/patient a break from discomfort during a treatment. Don't just plod on regardless of reactions (give relaxation treatment techniques). To continue to treat a sensitive foot for a longer period of time than the person can effectively cope with will result in there being too many toxins being released into the blood stream and this can result in making the client/patient feel ill and tired; completely defeating the object of the exercise.

CHILDREN

When dealing with children it is wise to make sure that the parent or guardian is aware of the limitations of the treatment. Never treat babies for longer than 5 minutes on the first session. This treatment should take the form of simple stroking upwards from heel to toe along all five zones, followed by light pressure on the reflex points of symptom areas. In general when dealing with children, treatment timings and pressures will vary according to the age of the child, the size of the child and symptoms presenting. The therapist will naturally have to use his/her judgement. The ultimate aim is to give all children a complete treatment using adjusted pressures.

When treating the very young it will often be sufficient to use only the index finger not the thumb. The therapist must use discretion with regard to timing when dealing with all clients, however this is even more important when dealing with children. - Children of all ages can benefit enormously from Reflexology.

It is important to note that it is a legal requirement as well as an ethical obligation to seek medical assistance for any undiagnosed conditions in children. Do not attempt to treat anything that may need medical attention.

THE ELDERLY

It might be necessary to take a little longer with these people. They cannot move quickly and while the therapist would naturally offer help where it is needed, it is not kind nor professional to rush the less able.

THE DIABETIC CLIENT (SEE PAGE 28 - 'CAUTION').
This condition requires careful treatment.

It is important for the therapist to keep to time as most people have busy schedules.

HOW TO DECIDE ON THE TREATMENT

All clients/patients should benefit from a course of eight treatments usually performed on a weekly basis (though this is not necessarily a requirement for all).

Many clients/patients like to maintain contact with the therapist on a monthly basis after the initial course.

Many clients/patients just require a 'one off' pick-me-up treatment.

All treatments should consist of a complete Reflexology routine with the exception of babies, the very young, the frail or those who require a symptomatic treatment due to a return visit in less than seven days. Details of treating certain clients/patients has been given on page 35-36. During the treatment routine when a reaction is felt the therapist should either stop and treat the specific reflex point again or alternatively make a mental note of the reflex and return and treat the area at the end of the normal routine.

If there appears to be **numerous** areas of sensitivity do not give extra treatment over and above the normal routine.

Many good therapists never break from this routine throughout their lives. It is a very good principle to which all student therapists should adhere.

Note!

Reflexology routines should not be mixed. In order to achieve the intended outcome maintain the routine of treatment designed by those who have the experience and knowledge so to do. Reflexology treatment is not a massage and should not be likened to massage.

REACTIONS TO REFLEXOLOGY (SECTION 1)

These can be broken into two types of reaction and the client/patient can have these reactions explained to them as part of the consultation.

1   Those reactions that happen during your treatment.

2   Those that happen after your treatment.

SOME OF THE REACTIONS THAT MIGHT HAPPEN DURING TREATMENT

A feeling of being very cold.
(Care should be taken not to give any heavy pressures and the circle pressures should be reduced to one or two; gradually increasing the number with successive treatments).

Changes in expression.

Crying, groaning, laughing, sighing or singing.

Gestures of pain.

Profuse sweating on the palms of the hands.

Visible contraction of the muscles.

To calm and relax the client/patient
Speak in a calm voice while gently effleuraging the whole foot. The effleurage can be alternated with a solar plexus massage or just stop and hold. For further information on how to deal with the above situations see page 187.

The therapist should also be aware that reactions unrelated to Reflexology could well occur in the clinic; for example, a heart attack or asthmatic attack. It is for this reason I think it necessary that all practising therapists should hold a valid Certificate in First Aid.

REACTIONS TO REFLEXOLOGY (SECTION 2)

REACTIONS OCCURRING BETWEEN TREATMENT SEQUENCES

These can sometimes involve temporary discomfort or pain.

Increase in urination.

Increase in bulk volume and frequency of the stool.

Increase in nasal secretions.

Increase of, or the appearance of, vaginal discharge.

Toothache, usually due to tooth decay or gum infections.

Feeling very tired.

Feeling very sleepy.

Feeling wonderful.

Clients/patients will also explain how, for example, they caught a cold last week after they had received a treatment. They will sometimes go on to express their fears of getting a cold etc., if they have more treatments. It is worthwhile taking the time to explain to the client/patient that all illness is preceeded by an incubation period which may last for days or much longer before the illness becomes apparent. Reflexology will not cause a cold. All reactions such as those described are due to the body's own healing and elimination processes.

All clients/patients who react in an unusual way or give the therapist grounds to suspect a serious illness must be referred to their own doctor. The therapist can always contact the client's doctor by letter explaining his/her fears (client's/patient's consent is required). The therapist may also ask the doctor for advice as to whether treatment can be continued or if it would be wiser to terminate the treatments during medical investigation. A sample of such a letter will be found on page 60.

Doctors may react in different ways to this type of letter both favourably and unfavourably. Some have been known to ask for a fee. However I am delighted to say that the majority of doctors I hear about are only too pleased to see therapists behaving in a caring and professional manner. All letters sent to a doctor which necessitate a reply should, as a matter of common courtesy, have a stamped addressed envelope enclosed.

The G.M.C.'s rules for doctors published in 'Professional Conduct and Discipline Fitness to Practice dated February 1991' (paragraph 42 & 43) allow a doctor to delegate to persons trained to perform special functions, treatment or procedures, provided that the **doctor** retains ultimate responsibility for the management of the patient.

The UK Government statement of December 3rd 1991 confirmed the doctor's right to delegate treatment of patients to specialists, including complementary therapist. Such treatment can be paid for by either the health authority or fund holding GP's.

PERSONAL HYGIENE

Take a daily bath or shower.

Prevent body odour by using a deodorant.

Use a mouthwash to prevent bad breath.

Clean teeth twice daily. Have regular dental checks.

Have a clean handkerchief in case of the necessity to cough or sneeze and please use it when necessary. Do not sneeze or cough over others.

Wear clean clothes and underwear daily.

Don't forget the socks, stockings or tights. They need changing at least once a day.

Keep hair clean and tidy. Make sure it does not fall onto your face when your head is bent as this can obscure the client's view; most people would prefer to see our faces when talking to us.

Keep nails short and, like the whole hand, impeccably clean.

Wash hands before and after each treatment.

Wash hands after using the toilet.

Wear a clean uniform or coat. It looks professional.

Wear clean shoes.

You must be able to take care of yourself before you attempt to take care of others.

You are offering a personal service where you are in very close proximity to others and your odour can be offensive to them. So if you smoke, drink or enjoy spicy food remember the smell can linger not just on your breath but on your clothes as well.

It is also worth bearing in mind that perfumes and aftershaves need to be used sparingly. The client might not share your love for a particular make or brand.

HYGIENE AT WORK

Hygiene is of the utmost importance in any treatment. When dealing with feet it is worth bearing in mind that the possibility of infection and contagion is always present. Conditions such as Athletes Foot (Tinea Pedis), Fungal infections of the nail and Verruca (a flat wart) are but a few.

1. The therapist's hands must be washed before and after each treatment.

2. A paper towel should be used to dry the feet.

3. Rest client's feet on a paper towel during treatment.

4. Cover knee and footrest with tissue. If tissue is not used then the covers must be changed after each client and washed before any further use.

5. Application of all solutions to the feet should be with cotton wool or tissue. A clean cotton wool or tissue to be used for each foot.

6. Sterilize bowl with liquid disinfectant after each use. All disposable material should be placed in a pedal bin immediately after use.

7. Have a pair of disposable gloves nearby for emergencies (athlete's foot requiring a closer examination).

8. Always read consultation card just prior to client's/patient's arrival to refresh your memory and always complete details of treatment on the card immediately the client/patient leaves or while he/she is getting ready to leave. Never put off this task until the end of the day or until you see "just one more client/patient".

9. At the end of the day waste should be burned if possible or placed in a plastic bag and sealed ready for refuse collection.

10. Make sure working area is clean and surroundings pleasant.

11. Do not smoke or allow client/patient to smoke during treatment.

THE THERAPIST AT WORK

Reflexology is an art. This art, like all other forms of art, will take time and a lot of practise to master. The student will soon realize this is not a subject that can be easily learned from a book. However, if it is not possible to receive tuition immediately, carefully following the instructions and diagrams in this book as well as paying special attention to the suggested routine should give the student adequate information for treating family members. I would, however, strongly advise all students thinking of working in the profession of Reflexology to take a qualifying course before working as a public practitioner (details at the end of this book).

Reflexology is not a cure for all ills, although this ancient therapy will help most people.

Before the treatment prepare a consultation card. (An example of such a card is given on page 55).

Check there are no contra-indications (reason why treatment cannot or should not be performed). There is a comprehensive list of precautions and contra-indications (pages 26 and 29).

Explain Reflexology to the client/patient. Keep it brief. Some people are very interested and will want to know more. In this case then, of course, do explain but do not fall into the trap of trying to explain all you know about the therapy at that moment. There is plenty of time during the treatment to chat.

When working it is necessary to use both hands; one to hold the foot or hand steady, the other to do the work.

Once again I have broken with tradition here and have not found it necessary to follow the theory or practice laid down by some, that it is obligatory to treat the left foot with the left hand and the right foot with the right hand. As a teacher I soon realized that not all my pupils were as dexterous as myself; so over the years I myself practised using my hands in all combinations imaginable and found the success of my treatments to be the same as when I performed the treatment using the corresponding hand. I now believe and teach that if the therapist finds working with one hand more comfortable than working with the other then he/she should work in this manner. Most Reflexology is performed using the basic thumb and finger technique. Work over the reflex area using the first joint of the thumb or finger not the whole digit. Many people believe that to use the inside or medial aspect of the digit is preferable to using the ball or tip. I personally do not subscribe to this theory.

The movement used in Reflexology is like bowing the first joint of the thumb or index finger up and down while making a slow movement over the reflex area. This movement has been likened to the movement of a caterpillar.

POSITION FOR WORKING

The comfort of both therapist and client is of equal importance for the completion of an enjoyable treatment. When the professional therapist works he or she uses the standard couch, porta-ped, or therapy chair, but if the treatment is being given in the home then an armchair can be used for the client but the client's lower legs and feet should be raised and supported. I have found that the padded adjustable garden chair (lounger) is the nearest to the ideal therapy chair.

In cold weather use a blanket to keep the client warm during treatment. A towel or two should be sufficient at other times.

The therapist should sit at a comfortable distance from the client's/patient's feet which should not necessitate the arms to be fully outstretched.

The treatment commences with a relaxing foot massage. It is during this massage that the therapist gets his/her first impression of the feet, noting temperature, colour, muscle and bone structure together with the condition of the skin.

It is important not to lay the client/patient flat. When working in the clinic situation use the couch/chair backrest for support. In the home or hospital situation place one or two cushions/pillows under the head. Both methods will enable the client/patient to see the therapist at work. This offers a measure of security and helps in building a relationship of trust. This position also gives the therapist the opportunity to observe the client's/patient's facial expressions and reactions, whether they be those of pain or relaxation, and therefore the treatment can be altered accordingly.

SOME JOINT LOOSENING EXERCISES TO PRACTISE BEFORE YOU START WORK

1   Stand with outstretched arms in front. Open and close hands ten times

2   Stand still holding arms outstretched as in the previous movement. Bend hand up and down from wrist ten times slowly, ten times fast.

3   Extend the arms to the side. Rotate wrist rapidly in a clockwise direction ten times. Repeat the movement in an anti-clockwise direction ten times.

4   Remain standing. Extend arms out to the side and push backwards twice. Bring arms to the front. Stretch out and push forward twice. Repeat complete movement ten times.

5   Stretch arms out in front, fingers pointing straight ahead, little finger side of hand towards floor, thumb toward ceiling. Hold fingers slightly apart. Now move hand from wrist up and down slowly at first gradually getting faster.

6   Stretch arms out in front. Close hand into fist, thumb on outside. Now throw your hands open. Repeat ten times.

7   Sit down and relax for a few minutes then bring your hands across in front of you. Close fingers into palm but leave thumb free. Try to make your thumbs bow to each other by bending the first joint (joint nearest nail). Repeat ten times.

8   Remain seated and this time try the movement by using your index finger (finger next to thumb) and remember to repeat ten times.

The next exercise to try is the Reflexology movement. Get a volunteer to let you practise on their feet. If there is not one around you can try this on your own hand.

1   Find the waist line area. Slide the thumb slowly across this line; lift and return to starting point.

2   This time move across in a slide-stop, slide-stop movement and then lift and return to start point.

3   Slide and stop as before only this time press ball and tip of thumb into foot (or hand). This will raise the first joint, (be careful not to dig your thumb nail into the flesh). Hold this position for a second, relax thumb and slide a fraction. Repeat movement. Continue this slide, press, raise until you reach the other side, then start all over again. Work thumb away from you if possible.

4   When you feel fairly confident with this movement using your thumb change to the index finger and repeat all of the movement in exactly the same way. Once again try to work moving index finger away from you all the time.

When you have mastered the art of bending the joint in the practise sessions across the foot, you can practise up and down the foot from heel to toe. Your aim is eventually to be able to walk across or up and down with little or no discomfort to you. Do not overdo this joint bending, as you might well have to pay the price the next day with aches and pains.

One other movement to practise is the webbing pinch. This is basically pinching between the toes. Place the index finger on top of the foot on the webbing and the thumb underneath the toes on the webbing. Grip the webbing between the fingers. A word of warning. This can be a very painful area so be very gentle.

The preceding movements are the main movements of Reflexology , however there are two further movements used by some therapists.

1. The Rotation. In this movement the thumb is placed on a painful area and the foot or hand is rotated.

2. The Hooking technique. The thumb is pressed very deeply into the flesh on the reflex point then used like a hook kept in place and the flesh pulled to one side. It is mainly used on the heel area due to the thickness of the flesh. **I personally do not like the hooking technique and feel no need for its use.**

IS IT NECESSARY TO GIVE A BOWL OF WATER?
IS IT NECESSARY TO USE OILS AND CREAMS?

Reflexology is a treatment always performed on clean feet. Offensive odour may cause embarrassment to both therapist and client alike. The client/patient will not relax and enjoy a treatment if they feel that you, the therapist, is being subjected to unpleasant smells or excessively sweaty feet.

It is a good idea to offer a bowl of water to those clients/patients who have not had a chance to take a shower or bath for some time. A building worker, for example, who has been in his shoes and socks all day is likely to sweat more than the average housewife. The water used should not contain chemical additives or perfume. A 5 ml of (1%) **pre-blended** Aromatherapy Oil (e.g. Lavender) or some Salt or Cider Vinegar is acceptable just to refresh. The water must not be hot as this will heat the feet artificially and as a result circulation will be increased. Further Reflexology may over stimulate and result in the treatment being less effective than it might otherwise be.

For those clients/patients who do not need a bowl of water the feet can be refreshed by wiping with a pad soaked in a refreshing solution i.e. Tonic, Witch Hazel or Surgical Spirit.

It is important to give a Reflexology Treatment on dry feet or hands. This gives the opportunity to feel and work deeply without the hands sliding over the flesh. It is for this reason I always dry the feet thoroughly after the cleaning or refreshing process. Some therapists like to use an Aromatherapy based cream, especially on dry or problem feet. I can see no reason why this cream cannot be applied at the end of the Reflexology part of the treatment and the final massage performed with it. Should the cream be used for the opening relaxation movements then it must be completely removed prior to the Reflexology treatment.

Note. Aromatherapy based cream should always be blended by a qualified Aromatherapist before being used by a Reflexologist. This cream must be in very low dilution ¼% to ½ % maximum.

The therapist is in a position to advise the client/patient of the benefits of bathing the feet daily and of the necessity to change socks or tights at least once a day in order to keep feet fresh and healthy. Exercise tact and thoughtfulness when giving such advice.

In the case of excessively sweaty feet the client should be advised to soak their feet as often as possible in a bowl of warm water to which has been added some lemon juice or vinegar. Better still would be to use 5 ml (1 teaspoon) of pre-blended Aromatherapy Essential Oil in the bath or foot bowl. These oils should be purchased from a professional Aromatherapist.

Note!
Excessively sweaty feet can benefit from regular Reflexology treatments. There are a number of recorded incidents where this problem has been successfully treated.

SECOND LAYER OF MUSCLES

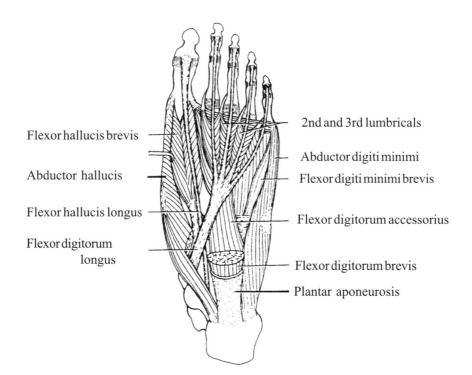

Flexor hallucis brevis

Abductor hallucis

Flexor hallucis longus

Flexor digitorum longus

2nd and 3rd lumbricals

Abductor digiti minimi

Flexor digiti minimi brevis

Flexor digitorum accessorius

Flexor digitorum brevis

Plantar aponeurosis

THE FIRST PAIR OF FEET

I HAVE NO ONE TO TEACH ME REFLEXOLOGY

Spend some time on the finger and thumb practise sessions (see page 47/49).

The first pair of feet are always the most frightening to begin work on. So the first thing to do is to learn client preparation, contra indications, precautions, hand exercise, the three transverse lines on the diagram, notes on hygiene and the foot massage.

Practise the foot relaxation movements on your own hand. This way at least you can learn the Step by Step routine which can remove some of the anguish when you come to a practical situation.

Find a friend or member of the family who would enjoy having a relaxing foot massage and would be patient while you practise your hand holds for giving the Reflexology treatment.

The first few practise sessions could be very simple and easy. There is no need at this stage to know which organ of the body is represented where on the foot; just follow these simple instructions and diagrams. When you have mastered this routine then it is time to progress to the full Reflexology routine.

Prepare the client with feet raised. Make yourself comfortable and begin.

When you have completed the relaxation treatment hold the foot steady with one hand and work with a Reflexology movement up and down all the toes underneath and on the sides using the free hand.

Next step is to use one hand to bend the toes back very gently and with the free hand (thumb) work from below the pad on the sole of the foot (diaphragm line - see diagram B -page 16) to the base of the toes. Cover the whole area, working upwards, returning to the diaphragm line each time. If you find it difficult to work up then work backwards and forwards across the area.

Move to the narrow part of the foot or waist line (see diagram B -page 16). Work up from the waist line to the diaphragm line in exactly the same manner as for the previous area. When you are satisfied that you have covered that area move down to the next line, the pelvic floor line, and repeat your movement from this line up to the waist line or across from Z 1 to Z 5.

Move down to tip of heel and work over the hard heel pad up to the pelvic floor line or across from Z 1 to Z 5. This movement can be alternated working from Z 5 to Z 1.

Lift the heel slightly and return it to rest in the palm of one of your hands. With the other hand stroke up the back and sides of the leg from heel to knee for as high as you can reach.

Next movement is to support the heel as before and with the thumb of the other hand work down the edge or side of the foot from the big toe to the heel, returning to start point and repeating the process (following the curve of the bone).

Change hands. This time work in the same manner but work from the edge of the foot on the little toe side to heel, returning to start point and repeating the process.

Work on toes on the top of the foot from nail to base; then work from base of toes towards the heel and the leg, work around the ankle area.

When working on the top and sides of the foot either work up and down or across the area whichever is more comfortable. The important thing is to have a method and a routine to follow.

A more specific professional routine for treatment commences on page 76 but do check page 64 for instructions on the introductory relaxation techniques. Remember these movements are important prior to the reflexology treatment.

Sample Consultation Card   CONFIDENTIAL

Name	Dr's Name
Address	Address
Tel No. H W	Tel No.
D.O.B	
Occupation	Height
Reason for Visit	Weight
Referred By	Date

Name and telephone number person who may be contacted in an emergency

Medical History

Medication to include Birth Control Pill or Hormone Replacement Therapy

Self prescribed medication (e.g. vitamin pills)

Illnesses : (Including those of childhood)

Operations

Accidents, injuries or falls with approximate dates

Back Problems

General State of Health

Do you or any member of your family suffer with any problems related to the following?
Diabetes, Epilepsy, Blood Pressure (H/L), Thrombosis, Heart, Chest, Migraine, Kidneys, Bladder, Digestion, Constipation, Colitis, Varicose Veins, Allergies, Hepatitis. Hay Fever, Asthma, M.S., Lupus, Cancer, Other.
Skin Problems.

Are you Pregnant?

Do you have regular Periods?

Date of last Period?

Do you suffer with Premenstrual Tension?   - What happens?

Last visit to Doctor. Reason?

Are you receiving any other therapy?

What therapy ?   Date of last treatment

Have you been to hospital for X-Ray or tests during the last three years?

Client's signature   Therapist

LIFE STYLES

DO YOU?

Smoke _____ How many daily _____

Drink alcohol _____Daily _____ Weekly _____ Infrequently _____

Drink   Tea _____ Coffee _____ How many daily _____

Drink   Water_____ How many glasses daily _____

Drink   Other liquids _____ How many glasses daily _____

Have a balanced diet _____ Eat regular meals _____

Eat before going to bed _____ Eat between meals _____

Take exercise _____Daily ____Weekly _____Infrequently____ Never_____

Work hours   Regular _____ Flexi _____ Shift _____ Unspecified ___

Take care of children _____How many _____Ages_____

Take care of the Elderly _____Sick _____ Handicapped _____

Sleep   Well _____ Poorly_____ Restlessly _____

Do you suffer from DEPRESSION/TENSION/ANXIETY/STRESS _____

How does the above condition affect you _____

_____

Is your outlook optimistic _____ pessimistic_____

Do you have any physical handicap _____

Do you wear glasses/contact lenses or hearing aid _____

POSTURE   Straight _____ Rounded shoulders _____

PERSONALITY   Confident _____ Nervous_____ Mixture _____

Do you live alone ?   Do you have a partner ?

Have you experienced a bereavement ?   If so when ?

	RIGHT FOOT	LEFT FOOT
Colour		
Skeletal Deformities		
Muscle Tone		
Flat Foot or High Arch		
Nail Condition		
Skin Condition		
Hard Skin Build up.		
Other		

THE REASON FOR THE CONSULTATION CARD

Through question and answer the therapist is able to ascertain if the client is suffering with any contagious or infectious conditions or indeed if there are any contra indications. A carefully recorded consultation card will help to build a picture of the client's/patient's general state of health and lifestyle. It is also giving the client/patient time to talk in a relaxed atmosphere and to get to know the therapist in a non threatening situation. It is during the consultation that the therapist is able to reassure the client/patient that all information shared with the therapist is completely confidential.

While the therapist should both ask the questions and complete the Consultation Card, the client's/patient's signature should be obtained on the completed card but not before he/she has been given the opportunity to read it.

The therapist can probe for more in depth answers and can learn a lot from the way in which the client/patient answers the questions.

Some people may not understand the terminology.

Remember some clients/patients cannot either read or write though they may well be verbally articulate.

THE TREATMENT CARD

This card gives the therapist the opportunity to record accurately, allowing him/ her to build a quick reference system as well as a complete picture of the client's/ patient's progress.

All therapists should keep accurate records of treatments. To make visual reference on a diagram or outline is helpful, but does not constitute accurate record keeping. Treatment card/sheet must be completed after each treatment and the case history summary should be completed after each course of treatments. It is a legal requirement that you keep accurate records for a minimum period of seven years.

A SAMPLE
TREATMENT CARD

Reactions since last treatment					
Date Time	R.F.	L.F.	Client Comments	Therapist's Coments	Therapist's Signature
16/5/96 10am	Sinuses C	Sinuses S	Very sensitive	Did not seem to relax	
Home Care advice given					

C = Crystal   S = Sensitivity   P = Pain   H = Hurt

The reverse of a treatment card can be used to build a case history of the client/ patient.

Case History
Summary/Evaluation

RENÉE TANNER
REFLEXOLOGIST
M. I. F. R.

Doctor S. Jones
11 Some Street
Croydon   1st June 1987

Dear Doctor Jones,
re: Mrs Mary Jane White, 00 Central Road, Croydon.

Your patient, my client, Mrs. M.J. White, has come to me for a Reflexology Treatment.

In view of the fact that she has had a recent operation and you are familiar with her condition, I would be grateful for your advice as to whether there is any medical reason why Mrs White should not receive Reflexology treatments at the present time. For your benefit I am enclosing an explanatory leaflet on the therapy, together with a copy of my professional membership certificate. Would you please sign the endorsement at the foot of this letter and with any comments, return it to me.

For your convenience I have enclosed a stamped addressed envelope for your reply together with a **signed consent form** from Mrs White giving me authority to request this information from you.

Yours faithfully,

Renée Tanner

78 Walkers Road, Croydon CR0 1OO   Tel:
....
I, Dr Jones can see no medical reason why Mrs Mary J White cannot receive a Reflexology Treatment.

Signed..

Dated..
Return to: Renée Tanner, 78 Walkers Road, Croydon CR0 1OO

THIRD LAYER OF MUSCLES IN THE SOLE

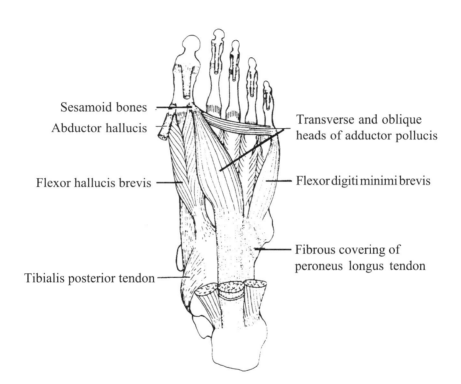

Sesamoid bones

Abductor hallucis

Flexor hallucis brevis

Tibialis posterior tendon

Transverse and oblique
heads of adductor pollucis

Flexor digiti minimi brevis

Fibrous covering of
peroneus longus tendon

A SUGGESTED METHOD FOR REFLEXOLOGY TREATMENT

1   Prepare client/patient consultation card and confirm as far as possible that there are no contra indications. Explain the treatment.

2   Examine feet

3   Cleanse and dry both feet

4   Give a relaxing foot massage to both feet - **Starting on right foot**

5   Perform reflexology treatment **- Starting on right foot**

6   Give a foot massage to both feet - **Starting on right foot**

7   Help the client/patient off the couch or out of the chair

8   Wash your hands

9   Make a further appointment if deemed to be necessary

10   Complete treatment record card

11   Prepare the couch for the next client/patient

12   Wash your hands again

TREATMENT TYPES

Two types of treatment are referred to in Reflexology

1. Symptomatic Treatment
2. Causal Treatment

Symptomatic treatment as the name suggests deals with the symptom. This is the type of treatment used in self help situations and by the therapist when a full treatment is inappropriate.
The way it works : - If someone has a pain in the head then the treatment is given to the reflex point of the head. Someone with stomach pains is treated only in the reflex area of the stomach.

Causal treatment is the type of treatment performed by the therapist seeking the underlying cause of the symptom. Therefore the entire foot receives a Reflexology treatment with the sensitive or crystal areas being given specific treatment over and above the normal routine.
For example the client complaining of headache might well be found to have a disorder in any of the five zones.
The client with stomach pains may be found to have reactions in the reflex areas of the stomach, intestines, lower back, solar plexus, etc.

In the main the qualified therapist will use Causal treatment. In other words the professional therapist working according to **this text book** treats zonal areas, reflex points and biological relationships, not just the reflex points related to the symptom.

MASSAGE / RELAXATION ROUTINE

PERFORMED PRIOR TO AND ON COMPLETION OF THE
REFLEXOLOGY ROUTINE

MASSAGE PRIOR TO AND ON COMPLETION OF A REFLEXOLOGY TREATMENT

Give client a bowl of warm water to soak feet, especially if he or she has been working all day. (This is a common courtesy to both client and therapist).

Alternatively, wipe feet with a cotton wool pad previously soaked in surgical spirit, witch hazel, proprietary antiseptic product, or similar solution.

1   Place both hands on top of the foot, fingers pointing towards ankle. Slide hands down foot from toes to ankle. Gently massage around ankle in large circular movements using two middle fingers.

2   Hold foot firmly, one hand under heel and place thumb of other hand on ball of foot just below toes. Fingers of this hand should be on top of foot. Rotate foot, first in clockwise movement then in an anti-clockwise movement. (Slow movement).

EFFLEURAGE (DIAGRAM REF. NO.1)

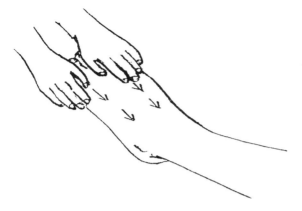

ROTATE (DIAGRAM REF. NO. 2)

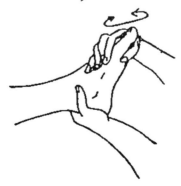

3   Put pad of hands (part below fingers = pad) on either side of foot, one on the medial aspect (big toe side) fingers pointing upwards (towards the leg). Push medial aspect from you with one hand while gently pulling the lateral aspect towards you with the other hand.
Repeat in the opposite direction, pushing lateral aspect away while gently pulling the medial aspect towards you.

4   Place fingers on top of foot, thumbs underneath. Have balls of thumb flat against sole, fingers flat on top (one hand will be lower down the foot than the other). Work thumbs in a zig-zag movement from base of toes to base of heel and back up to the base of the toes (quick movement).

PUSH PULL (DIAGRAM REF. NO. 3)

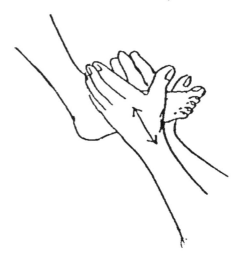

ZIG ZAG (DIAGRAM REF. NO.4)

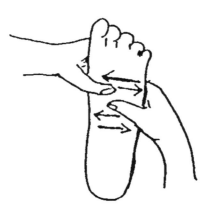

5   Place both hands on top of the foot, fingers pointing towards ankle. Slide hands down foot from toes to ankle. Gently massage around ankle in large circular movements using two middle fingers.

6   Hold foot with one hand. With heel of other hand give a deep firm stroke down inner aspect (big toe side) from toe to heel. Keep had on side of foot not sole.

Note. Follow the curve of the bone. Do not work straight down as this will over treat the bladder reflex.

ANKLE MASSAGE (DIAGRAM REF. NO. 5)

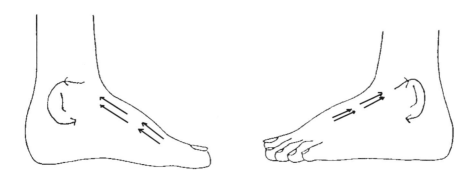

HEEL OF HAND DOWN INSIDE FOOT
(DIAGRAM REF. NO. 6)

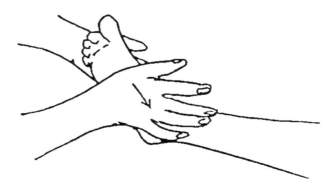

7   Put pad of hands (palm) on either side of foot, one on the medial aspect (big toe side) fingers pointing upwards (towards the leg). Push medial aspect from you with one hand while gently pulling the lateral aspect towards you with the other hand.
Repeat in the opposite direction, pushing lateral aspect away while gently pulling the medial aspect towards you.

8   Hold foot firmly, one hand under heel and place other hand with thumb on ball of foot just below toes. Fingers of this hand should be on top of foot. Rotate foot, firstly in a clockwise movement then in an anti-clockwise movement. (Slow movement).

PUSH PULL (DIAGRAM REF. NO. 7)

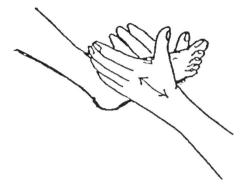

ROTATE (DIAGRAM REF. NO. 8)

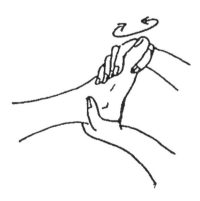

9 Place hands in position as for movement number 4. Slide down sole to heel. Firmly grip foot and pull upwards from heel towards toes, (all pulling pressure is on sole not top of foot, as this would hurt). Spread toes gently. Put hand on top of toes and then slide fingers from toe to toe, parting toes and then allowing them to fall back into place.

10 Hold toes with one hand and bend them away from you (just a little); place the thumb of the free hand in position just below the ball of the foot on the medial edge (just beneath the ball of the big toe). It should be pointing towards the little toe with the inner aspect touching the ball of the foot. With a caterpillar like movement work across the foot towards the little toe (along the diaphragm line). Repeat this movement. However if your hands are supple or you are naturally left handed, then you could change hands and work in the opposite direction.

PULL UP HEEL TO TOE, SPREAD TOES
(DIAGRAM REF. NO. 9)

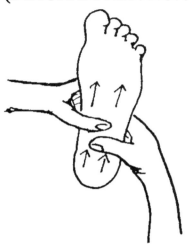
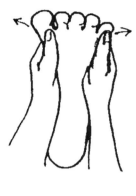

DIAPHRAGM LINE
(DIAGRAM REF. NO. 10)

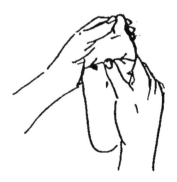

BONES OF THE FOOT

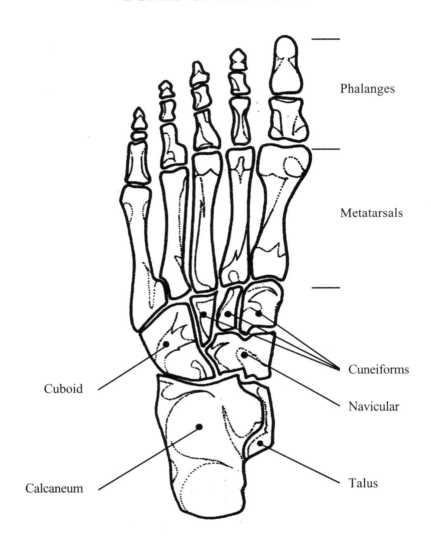

Phalanges

Metatarsals

Cuneiforms

Cuboid

Navicular

Calcaneum

Talus

REFLEXOLOGY ROUTINE

RIGHT FOOT

TREATMENT ON RIGHT FOOT

1. DIAPHRAGM / SOLAR PLEXUS
Z 1 TO Z 5 AND Z 2/3

Gently push all the toes backwards with one hand. This will make the diaphragm line more visible. While holding this position use thumb of free hand to work along the diaphragm line from Z 1 to between Z 2 and Z 3 solar plexus. Stop at this point turn thumb so tip is pointing towards the toes and press three times . Then continue to work across the foot on diaphragm line to Z 5. Then repeat the entire process.

2. HEAD AND BRAIN
Z 1 TOE ONE

Work with the thumb from the base of the big toe (outside edge) up the outside, over the top and down the inner side (in a horseshoe shape). Return to the start point and repeat the movement. **Return** to the start point again, only this time work from the base of the big toe underneath to the top. Continue this movement until the base area of the big toe is treated (X 2). Now work on the top of the toe in a similar way; only this time work from the **bottom of the nail down** to the bottom of the toe (area where toe joins foot). Make sure to treat the whole area of the top of the toe X 2.

Areas of the Toe
Treatment of the upper part of the toe area is covering the whole face (eyes, nose, mouth, jaws, gums, and teeth).

Treatment over the top and sides of the toe is covering the brain, cranial nerves, sides of the head and ears.

Treatment on the base of the toe (sole) is covering the back of the head including the systems connected with it (bones, muscles, nerves, blood supply, brain etc.)

DIAPHRAGM / SOLAR PLEXUS

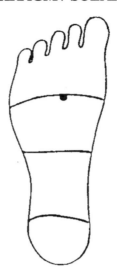

HEAD AND BRAIN

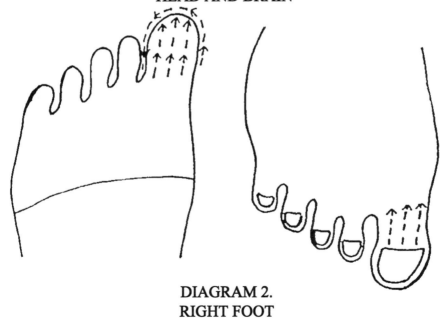

DIAGRAM 2.
RIGHT FOOT

3.   FRONT OF NECK/GENERAL NECK
Z 1 TOE ONE

Put index finger at the base of the big toe; on top of the foot. Work across this base line from the outside of the toe to the inside. Stop between toe 1 and toe 2. Then return to start point and repeat the movement X 2. Making a total of three movements.

Treatment of this area is covering all the structures of the neck/throat, thyroid, parathyroid, tonsils, epiglottis, vocal cords, eustachian tubes (reactions in the lymph tissue of the tonsil is found on the side of the big toe at its base next to Z 2). There is also a very small point on the median line at the base of the great toe on the neck reflex that will sometimes react when the tonsil is energy starved.

4.   BACK OF NECK
Z 1 TOE ONE

Work in a straight line across the base crease of the big toe (underneath). Start from outside edge. Work to inside (between toe 1 and toe 2). Return to start point and repeat X 2.

Treatment of this area is covering muscular and skeletal structures of the neck as well as all the points found in the front of the neck area.

Note. The base of the toe is very small therefore all the structures of the neck are to be found in both the front and back. However experience has proven that certain areas react more favourably on one side than the other.

FRONT OF NECK

**DIAGRAM 3
RIGHT FOOT**
(Top)

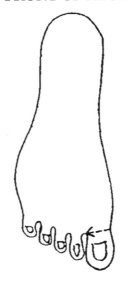

BACK OF NECK

**DIAGRAM 4
RIGHT FOOT**
(Sole)

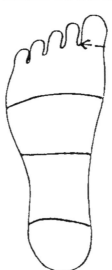

5. OCCIPITAL

Z 1 TOE ONE

Use thumb to caterpillar walk up the base of the big toe close to the inside edge.
Start the movement from the base crease line (neck area) and make 3 very small
movements up towards the top of the toe. Stop and give 3 definite presses.

Note. This movement is performed on the base (sole) of the toe not the inner
side.

6. EAR POINT / MASTOID PROCESS

Z 1 TOE ONE

Work up toe from occipital point 1 further movement to the mastoid process.
Give 3 definite presses.

6A. TEMPLE

Work up from the mastoid area for two small points to just below the crown of
the top of the toe. Give three definite presses.

OCCIPITAL

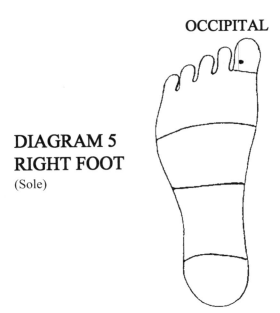

DIAGRAM 5
RIGHT FOOT
(Sole)

EAR POINT - MASTOID PROCESS

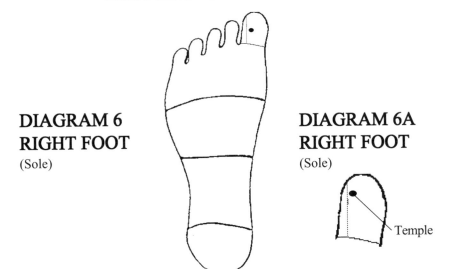

DIAGRAM 6
RIGHT FOOT
(Sole)

DIAGRAM 6A
RIGHT FOOT
(Sole)

Temple

7. PITUITARY

Z 1 TOE ONE

Place thumb in centre of pad on the big toe (sole) pointing towards the top of the toe. Press X 3.

Note. When treating a client who suffers from Acne type skin or if there are any problems related to the endocrine system in general press and release X 3 again.

7A. PINEAL GLAND \ HYPOTHALAMUS

Place the thumb on the pituitary gland, move one very small point up towards the top of the toe. Rock the thumb over onto its outer edge and give three pressure type circles (using the outer edge of the thumb). Without lifting the thumb, rock the thumb over onto its inside edge and give three pressure type circles using the inside edge of the thumb.

Note.   Neither set of pressure circles will be given directly on to the pituitary gland but **just** above it.

8. SINUSES / CRANIAL NERVES

Z 2 TO Z 5. FOUR TOES

Work with the index finger from the base of the side of toe (between toe 1 and toe 2) up the side of toe two over the top and down the other side in a horseshoe shape. Repeat as on the big toe. Next work with the thumb from the base of the toe (underneath) to the top of the toe X 1. Work once more from the base of toe to the bulb, push the bulb up and gently backwards, as if trying to roll it over the top of the toe. Treat all toes 2 to 5. Repeat on each toe 1 to 5.

Note.   The area of the cranial nerves will be found on the sides of the toes.

Note.   Where sinus problems or headaches exist repeat the entire movement (No.8) once more.

PITUITARY

**DIAGRAM 7
RIGHT FOOT**
(Sole)

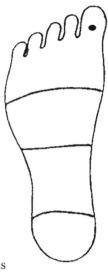

**DIAGRAM 7A
RIGHT FOOT**
(Sole)

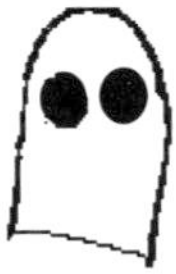

Pineal
& Hypothalamus

SINUSES

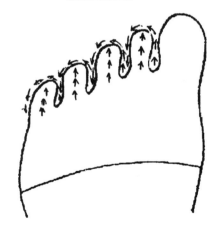

**DIAGRAM 8
RIGHT FOOT**
(Sole)

9.   TEETH
Z 1 TO Z 5. FIVE TOES

This time work on top of the toes. Start at the base of the nail and work down to the bottom of each individual toe X 2. Do as many movements as are necessary to cover the whole width of the toe from nail to base.

Note   All teeth are treated on the big toe in general
        Incisors and Canine teeth   toe 2
        Premolars   toe 3
        Molars   toe 4
        Wisdom   toe 5

10. LYMPHATICS OF HEAD / NECK
Z 1 TO Z 5 BETWEEN TOES

Very gently pinch webbing between toes.

Note. When treating webbing between Z 1 and Z 2 especially against the base of the big toe a reaction may be noted. This area represents the tonsils helper.

TEETH

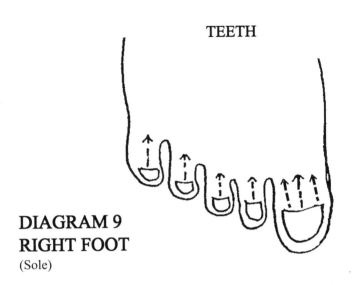

DIAGRAM 9
RIGHT FOOT
(Sole)

LYMPHATICS OF HEAD / NECK

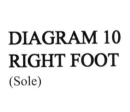 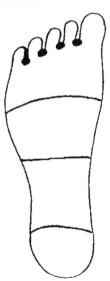

DIAGRAM 10
RIGHT FOOT
(Sole)

11.   EYES / EARS
Z 2 TO Z 5 UNDER TOES

Bend toes back gently. With thumb of free hand work on top part of exposed pad along the top of the ridge at the base of the toes. Work from Z 2 to Z 5 X 2.
Note. **Eyes** under Z 2/3 and **ears** under Z 4/5.
Remember that while working across this ridge pressure will in the main be in a downward movement with the medial aspect (inner side) of the thumb pressing against the base of the toes. It is also worth noting that sometimes there will be a reaction felt at the base of toe three (just above the metatarsophalangeal joint) when there is an energy blockage to the ear. This will always be confirmed when treating the ear area in Z 4 and Z 5.

12.   EYE POINT (MAJOR HELPER)
Z 2/3 UNDER TOES

Use thumb or index finger to press down firmly on the pad at the base of the toes (sole) between Z 2 and Z 3 (do not press into toes).

Note.   This is a major helper reflex point to the eye, often reacting in people who normally wear contact lenses.

Note.   A further reaction is sometimes felt at the base of toe 2 (just above the metatarsophalangeal joint) when there is an energy blockage to the eye. This will always be confirmed when treating the eye area between Z 2 and Z 3. The eye, like all the face, is also treated on the great toe.

EYES / EARS

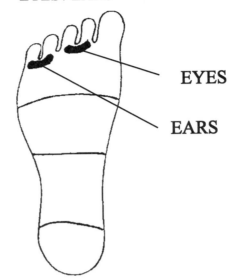

EYES

EARS

**DIAGRAM 11
RIGHT FOOT**
(Sole)

EYE POINT - Major Helper

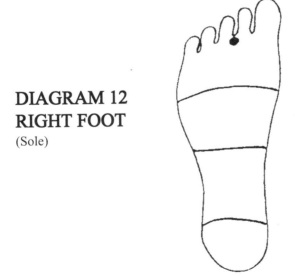

**DIAGRAM 12
RIGHT FOOT**
(Sole)

13. EAR POINT (MAJOR HELPER)
Z 4/5 UNDER TOES

Use thumb or index finger to press down firmly on the pad at the base of toes (sole) between Z 4 and Z 5 (Do not press into toes). This is a major reflex point for the ear often reacting in people who have has their ear syringed or in those who suffer with a wax problem.

Note. While this is a major reflex helper to the ear it should be remembered that the ear is also treated on the big toe and toe 3 with reflex points too small to be identified by all but the most experienced therapists. Middle ear problems often react on toe 3.

14. EUSTACHIAN TUBE
Z 3/4/ UNDER TOES

Put the index finger of one hand at the base of the toes between Z 3 and Z 4 on the top of the foot. Put the thumb of the same hand on the sole at the base of the toes (on the pad) between Z 3 and Z 4. Push down firmly towards the heel while pinching together gently. This hold is on the fleshy area not on or between the toes.

Note. This is a helper reflex point for the eustachian tube. Eustachian tube also treated on the big toe.

EAR POINT -Major Helper

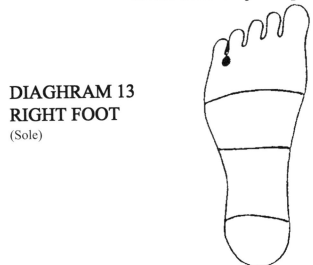

**DIAGHRAM 13
RIGHT FOOT**
(Sole)

EUSTACHIAN TUBE

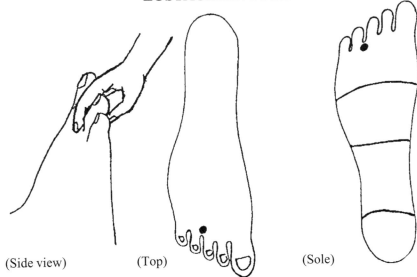

(Side view)   (Top)   (Sole)

**DIAGRAM 14
RIGHT FOOT**

15. BALANCE

Z 4 TOE FOUR

Slide index finger down top of toe 4 from base of nail to base of toe; then press into base X 2.

16. SHOULDER POINT / LYMPHATICS
Z 4/5 TOP OF FOOT AND SOLE

Use index finger to slide down from the base of the toes (top of foot) between toe 4 and toe 5 to just below the knuckle area (metatarsophalangeal joint). Put the thumb on the corresponding point on the sole area of the foot, press firmly X 2. **Hold the thumb and finger in the grip position, allow hand to fall to the side and work with seven circular movements while maintaining the grip.**

Note.   Fingers and thumb should not slide over the flesh for this movement but should be held in position while the flesh is moved. This action should mimic that of shoulder rotation

BALANCE

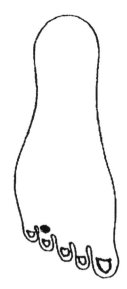

DIAGRAM 15
RIGHT FOOT
(Top)

SHOULDER POINT

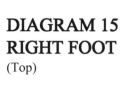

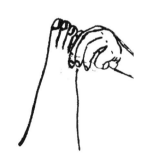

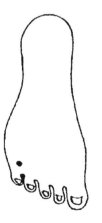

(Outer side)

DIAGRAM 16
RIGHT FOOT

Top

17. THYROID / PARATHYROID / THYMUS
(general area helper) (ZONAL)

Z 1 SOLE

Place the thumb on the diaphragm line at the outer edge of Z 1 toe 1. Begin caterpillar like walk towards Z 2 but stop between Z 1 and Z 2. Turn the thumb to point towards the toes and work up crease line to between big toe and toe 2. Return to start point and repeat entire movement.

17A. THYROID (ZONAL)

Z 1 SOLE

Lift the thumb and place it in the centre of the pad of the ball of the foot Z 1. Move one point up towards the base of the big toe and give three pressure circles.

THYROID / PARATHYROID / THYMUS / BRONCHI / TRACHEA (GENERAL AREA TREATMENT)

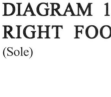

DIAGRAM 17
RIGHT FOOT
(Sole)

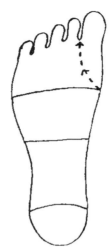

THYROID

DIAGRAM 17A
RIGHT FOOT
(Sole)

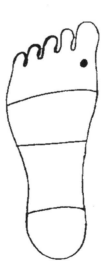

17B.   PARATHYROID (ZONAL)

Z 1 SOLE

Lift the thumb and place it in line with the thyroid on the edge of zone one (next to Z 2); move thumb one point up towards the base of the big toe and give three pressure circles.

17C.   THYMUS (ZONAL)

Z 1 SOLE

Lift the thumb and place it in line with the thyroid, move one tiny point down and one tiny point out towards the edge of the foot (as close to the edge of the foot as possible while still working on the sole). Give three pressure circles.

18. OESOPHAGUS / TRACHEA

Z 1 SOLE

Place the thumb on the diaphragm line at the edge of Z 1 (medial aspect of foot). Work from this point up to the base of the big toe. Return to diaphragm line and continue to work to base of toe until the entire pad has been treated in this way.

Note. Two thirds of this area represents the oesophagus (working from edge of foot towards Z 2) the other third represents the trachea. Two points up from the diaphragm line the trachea/bronchi (area one third closest to Z 2) enter the lungs.

Also note that on Z 1 working up for 1 point from diaphragm lies the reflex area for a hiatus hernia. (See diagram opposite)

95

PARATHYROID

DIAGRAM 17B
RIGHT FOOT
(Sole)

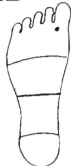

THYMUS

DIAGRAM 17C
RIGHT FOOT
(Sole)

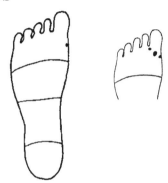

OESOPHAGUS / TRACHEA

DIAGRAM 18
RIGHT FOOT
(Sole)

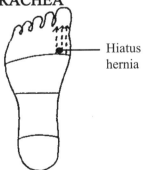

Hiatus
hernia

19. CHEST / LUNGS / SHOULDER
Z 2 TO Z 5 SOLE

Put thumb on diaphragm line directly under Z 2 (edge of Z 1). Work from diaphragm line to base of toes. Continue to work in this manner until the entire area from Z 2 to Z 5 has been treated. Repeat movement.

Note. When working from diaphragm line Z 5 to base of toe 5 reactions will give indications of shoulder reflex not lungs. Reactions occuring between Z 2 and Z 4 indicates lungs

Note. Exercise caution in this area if a pace maker is fitted.

19A. SHOULDER GIRDLE / SCAPULA

On the sole of the foot just below the toes is a ridge prominence. One tiny point below this ridge Z 1 to Z 5 is the reflex point for the shoulder girdle, scapula and clavicle.

Note. This area is treated with number 19 and is thus not treated again unless a reaction is felt. Should a reaction be felt then this area should be treated separately as follows :- Work across the reflex from Z 1 to Z 5 X 2.

20. CHEST / LUNGS CONTINUED
Z 1 TO Z 5 TOP OF FOOT

This time work on top of the foot and use the index finger and not the thumb. Start at the base of the big toe and work with caterpillar movements down the foot towards the ankle, to a point corresponding to the diaphragm line. Treat all five zones in this manner. When the area has been treated return to the start point and repeat the process.

Note. This area is also treating the ribs and general musculature of the chest

CHEST / LUNGS

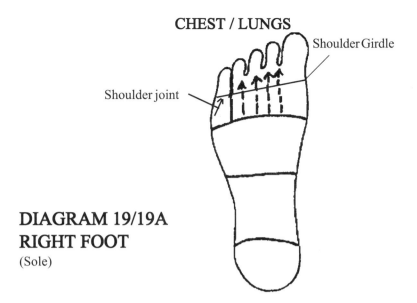

Shoulder Girdle

Shoulder joint

DIAGRAM 19/19A
RIGHT FOOT
(Sole)

CHEST / LUNGS - CONTINUED

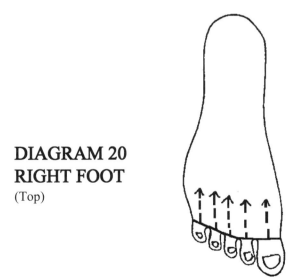

DIAGRAM 20
RIGHT FOOT
(Top)

21. UPPER ABDOMEN

Z 1 TO Z 5 SOLE

Do not treat this area if a heart monitor/support device box is fitted within this area.

Put thumb on diaphragm line Z 1 as close to the edge of the foot as possible. Work across the foot from Z 1 to Z 5. Continue to work in this manner until the entire area between diaphragm line and waist line has been treated. Return to start point and repeat movement.

Note. Just above the waist line on Z 1 (see diagram) is found the reflex point for the Pyloric Sphincter

22. GALL BLADDER (RIGHT FOOT ONLY)

BETWEEN Z 3/4 SOLE

Place the thumb on the upper abdomen the tip touching the diaphragm line between Z 3 and Z 4. Press X 2.
Use all of the first joint of the thumb (distal joint) for this pressure

Note. Treat very gently over area if gall stones are present.

UPPER ABDOMEN

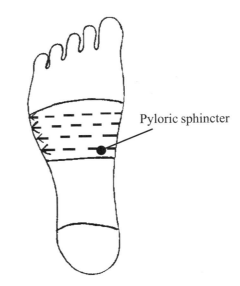

**DIAGRAM 21
RIGHT FOOT**
(Sole)

Pyloric sphincter

GALL BLADDER

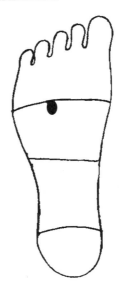

**DIAGRAM 22
RIGHT FOOT**
(Sole)

23. LIVER (RIGHT FOOT ONLY)
Z 3 TO Z 5 SOLE

Place the thumb on Z 3 just under the diaphragm line pointing towards Z 5. Work from Z 3 to Z 5 for three straight but slightly overlapping rows (each new row commencing slightly further down the foot from the previous one). Change hands. This time work as before but from Z 5 to Z 3. It is worth remembering that if difficulties are being experienced changing hands to work in opposite direction, then work in one direction only (repeat movement).

Note. The main reflex for the liver is treated between Z 3 and Z 5. However the liver does extend across towards zone 1 and even onto part of Z 1 on the left foot. The entire liver benefits by being treated with the upper abdomen while the major reflex point is given specific treatment on the right foot only.

24. STOMACH / PANCREAS / DUODENUM
Z 1 TO Z 2 SOLE

Do not treat this area if a heart monitor/support device box is fitted within this area.

Place the thumb just below diaphragm line on the sole close to the median line (to the edge of the foot). By placing the thumb flat on the sole with the inner edge against the diaphragm line you will be in the correct place to commence. Work from Z 1 to Z 2 across the foot in three straight but slightly overlapping rows. On completion of the three rows repeat the movement in the opposite direction. If experiencing difficulty in changing hands or working in the opposite direction then return to start point and repeat the movement as before.

Line 1   Stomach (Cardia Sphincter)
Line 2   Pancreas / Duodenum
Line 3   Duodenum

Exercise great care when dealing with a diabetic or a client who is suffering stomach ulcers (work very gently).

LIVER

DIAGRAM 23
RIGHT FOOT
(Sole)

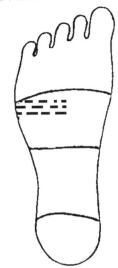

STOMACH / PANCREAS / DUODENUM

DIAGRAM 24
RIGHT FOOT
(Sole)

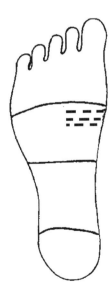

25. LOWER ABDOMEN / SMALL INTESTINE
Z 1 TO Z 5 SOLE

Put thumb on waist line, work with caterpillar like movement from Z 1 to Z 5 until entire area between waist line and pelvic floor line has been treated. Repeat movement in opposite direction i.e. Z 5 to Z 1.

Important Note - Though some therapists work this area upwards (longitudinal) my experience has shown that the recipient has a tendency to feel sick. I have proven to my own satisfaction that to work across the foot gives better results.

25A LOWER BACK \ PELVIS \ SCIATIC
(general zonal helper area)
Z 1 TO Z 5

Put the thumb on the hard heel pad just below the pelvic floor line. Work with caterpillar like movements across the foot from Z 1 to Z 5. Treat entire heel pad area. When area has been treated in this direction then caterpillar walk upwards on each zone from base of heel to pelvic floor line (treat entire heel pad area). Do not repeat this movement

26. SCIATIC LINE
UP BACK OF LEG

Put one hand under leg, palm uppermost (against leg). Then with a slow, sliding type, push movement, work from ankle up to behind the knee; return to the start point and repeat X 2. Return to start point again, this time close heel of hand onto leg in a squeezing movement. Work up leg to behind knee. Return to start point and repeat X 2.

LOWER ABDOMEN / PELVIS / SMALL INTESTINE

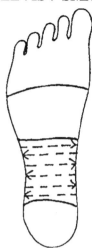

**DIAGRAM 25
RIGHT FOOT**

SCIATIC LINE

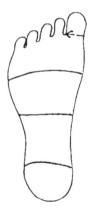

**DIAGRAM 26
RIGHT FOOT**

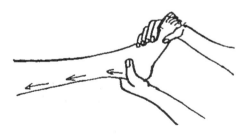

**DIAGRAM 25A
RIGHT FOOT**

27. SCIATIC LINE - CONTINUED
BEHIND ANKLE - ACROSS SOLE

Put thumb of one hand (pointing down towards the sole) on the soft flesh area behind the ankle bone at its highest point. Work with caterpillar like movements down behind ankle bone then across the hard heel pad on the sole of the foot (change hands if necessary) and continue to work with this movement up behind the other ankle bone to its highest point. Return to start point and repeat movement X 2. (Total of three).

Note. On hard heel pad (sciatic line) between Z 3/4 there is likely to be a reaction when sciatic problems exist. Treat in usual manner with pressure circles.

28. SPINE
INNER EDGE OF FOOT

Use the thumb to work with caterpillar like movements down inner edge of foot (medial aspect) from just below nail area on big toe to the heel. Follow the curve of the foot (feeling for the bone). Repeat movement in opposite direction from heel to toe, then repeat entire movement. Do not work straight up and down as this will cross and overstimulate the bladder (see diagram P 104)

Note. Due to the huge supply of nerves directly from the spinal cord to the organs and structures of the body, treating the spine works not only on the skeletal and muscular structure of the area but gives a general treatment to the other organs and structures of the body.

SCIATIC LINE - CONTINUED

DIAGRAM 27
RIGHT FOOT

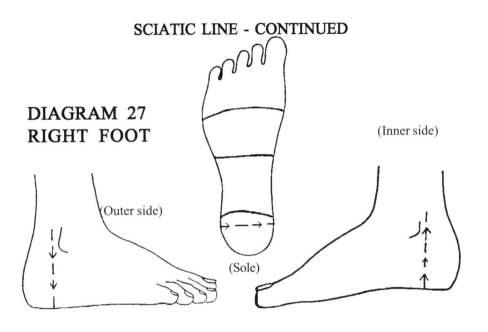

(Outer side)

(Inner side)

(Sole)

SPINE

DIAGRAM 28
RIGHT FOOT
(Sole Inner side)

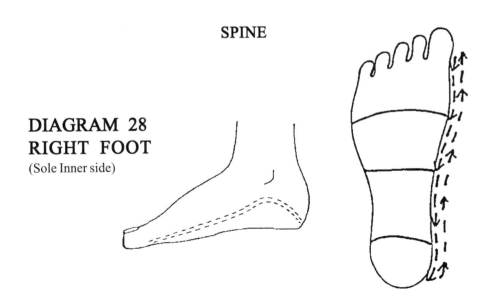

29. SHOULDER / ELBOW / KNEE / HIP / LOWER BACK
OUTER EDGE OF FOOT

Use the thumb to work with caterpillar like movement down outer edge of the foot from below nail area on little toe to the heel. (first three walks are treating the shoulder reflex) Repeat entire movement in opposite direction then repeat the entire movement again

29A ELBOW HELPER

Caterpillar walk down outer edge of foot for four points (2 points below the 5th metatarsophalangeal joint) turn thumb and caterpillar walk on to the top of the foot for three points, then give three pressure circles.

29B KNEE HELPER

Immediately the protrusion on the side of the foot is felt (base of the fifth metatarsal) caterpillar walk on to the top of the foot for five points. Give three pressure circles. When a knee problem exists and no sign of energy blockage is evident turn the thumb and work up towards the toes on a level with the elbow reflex. Press X 5

29C HIP HELPER

Caterpillar walk from the end of the protrusion (end nearest heel) in a diagonal line to the base of the ankle. Change hands and caterpillar walk down from the base of the ankle in a straight line to the edge of the heel. Caterpillar walk up from the edge of the foot to the base of the ankle to fill in the gap in the triangle.

30. RECTUM / ANUS / LOWER PELVIS
Z 1 TO Z 5

Put thumb on outer edge of heel in line with ankle (pointing towards the floor with the fingers resting on the sole of the foot). Work with caterpillar movement around behind the heel to the corresponding point on the opposite side which is just one point below the bladder reflex. Stop and give three pressure circles on this reflex area of the rectum/anus return to start point and repeat the movement. **Note.** This movement is completed in a horseshoe shape, it may be commenced from medial aspect (inner side of the foot) or the lateral aspect (outside of foot). Just remember to give three pressure circles on the rectum/anus helper point (inner side of foot)

SHOULDER / ELBOW / KNEE / HIP / LOWER BACK

**DIAGRAM 29
RIGHT FOOT**
(Sole)

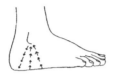

**DIAGRAM 29C
RIGHT FOOT**

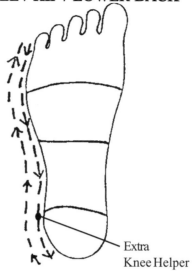

Extra
Knee Helper

RECTUM / ANUS LOWER PELVIC POINT

**DIAGRAM 30
RIGHT FOOT**
(Sole)

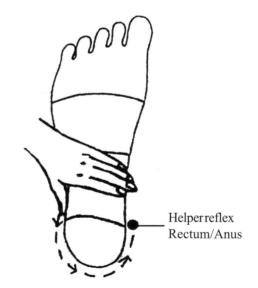

Helper reflex
Rectum/Anus

31. KIDNEY / URETER TUBES

Place thumb to straddle the waist line between Z 2 and Z 3. Use left hand on right foot. With tip of thumb pointing towards toes press and release X 2. Remove thumb, replace thumb and press and release X 2 again. Swivel thumb around so that the tip of the thumb is pointing towards heel, work down the ureter tubes (Z 2) along the side of the tendon to the hard heel pad. Twist hand around, still using thumb, walk up the side of the foot (medial aspect) to centre of the bladder (between three and four points/walks up onto side of foot) press X 3 (bladder usually is a slightly puffy area on the inside of the foot). See number 32 for information on the bladder.

32. BLADDER

INNER SIDE OF FOOT

The bladder is usually visible as a slightly puffy area between three and four points/walks up onto the medial aspect of the foot proximal to the pelvic floor line (big toe side - see diagram) Place the thumb in the centre of the bladder area then work in points radiating outwards. (Use three small caterpillar like movements for 4 lines).

Do not work back up ureter tubes towards kidney as this may transfer any infection present in the bladder to the kidney. To treat in this way would work against the way nature has designed the system to work.

KIDNEY / URETER TUBES

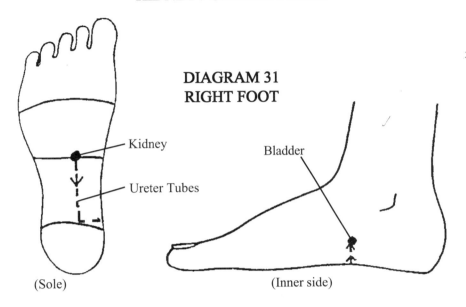

DIAGRAM 31
RIGHT FOOT

Kidney

Ureter Tubes

Bladder

(Sole)

(Inner side)

BLADDER

DIAGRAM 32
RIGHT FOOT
(Sole)

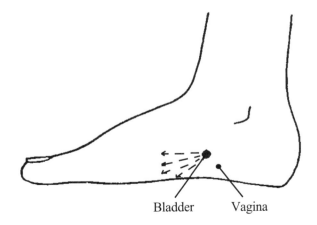

Bladder   Vagina

110

33. ADRENALS

Z 1/2

Put one thumb on the kidney point pointing towards toes and bring second thumb to meet it (on the big toe side). This thumb should be pointing towards the heel. Now both thumbs should be pointing in opposite directions with nails almost parallel. Remove the thumb from the kidney point. With the remaining thumb on the adrenal gland press and release gently X 3. If client/patient suffers with acne type skin or there are any problems related to the endocrine system then press this area a further three times.

34. UTERUS / PROSTATE

BELOW INNER ANKLE

Place index finger on inner ankle bone.
Place third finger on tip of heel.
Bend second finger slightly, it will fall in line with the other fingers. When the point of importance has been located by middle finger, remove all three fingers and place the thumb on point where the middle finger rested. Press and release X3.
This location movement can be performed with the index finger on the heel and the third finger on the ankle bone if this is found to be a more comfortable position for the therapist.
Note. If IUD is fitted work with great care and do not press directly on to the uterus area but gently stroke over the area with the two middle fingers

111

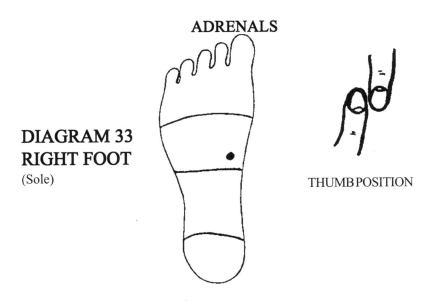

ADRENALS

**DIAGRAM 33
RIGHT FOOT**
(Sole)

THUMB POSITION

UTERUS / PROSTATE

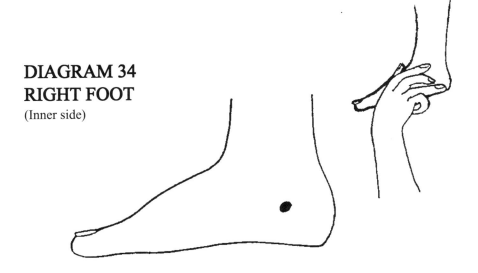

**DIAGRAM 34
RIGHT FOOT**
(Inner side)

35. OVARIES / TESTES

BELOW OUTER ANKLE

Place index finger on outer ankle bone.

Place third finger on tip of heel.

Bend second finger slightly, it will fall in line with the other fingers. When the point of importance has been located by middle finger, remove all three fingers and place the thumb on point where the middle finger rested. Press and release X3.

This movement can be performed with the index finger on the heel and the third finger on the ankle bone if this is found to be a more comfortable position for the therapist.

Note. If the client suffers from acne type skin or if there are any problems related to the endocrine system repeat the pressure X 3 again.

36. FALLOPIAN TUBES / VAS DEFERENS

TOP OF FOOT

Work with caterpillar like movement from outer ankle to inner ankle across crease line between foot and leg. Repeat this movement x 2.

OVARIES / TESTES

DIAGRAM 35
RIGHT FOOT
(Outer side)

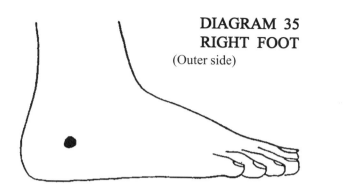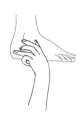

FALLOPIAN TUBES / VAS DEFERENS

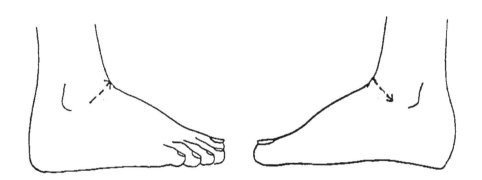

DIAGRAM 36
RIGHT FOOT

37. LYMPHATIC / INGUINALS / PELVIC AREA

Place the thumb on the outer edge of the heel (see diagram) pointing upwards towards the leg.

Work up behind the ankle to an area one point higher than the ankle bone, press and release X 2. Then pull slide the thumb back to the bottom of the ankle and work around the base of the bone and up in front of the ankle bone (horseshoe shape) press X 2 one point higher than the ankle bone. Slide the thumb back to the base of the bone, turn the thumb and work across the leg-foot crease line to the other ankle. Change hands and repeat the whole process on the other ankle. Commence at the beginning again and repeat the movement on both ankles.
Note. This movement may be commenced on either ankle. Ensure both ankles are treated twice.

38. BREAST AREA
Z 2 TO Z 5 TOP OF FOOT

Use pad of index finger to work on the top of the foot in a gentle, slow, slide, press and release movement from the base of the toes to an area corresponding to the diaphragm line on the sole. Start movement at the base of toe 2. Work down Z 2, work back using a gentle pull and press movement. Work each zone 2 to 5 in this manner. This movement should be superficial.
Note. Return movement is almost like caterpillar walk in reverse.
It is important to remember that when working between the metatarsals the musculature of the chest are being treated as well as the more superficial breast. The ribs are represented by the metatarsals.

CHANGE TO LEFT FOOT

LYMPHATICS / INGUINALS / PELVIC AREA

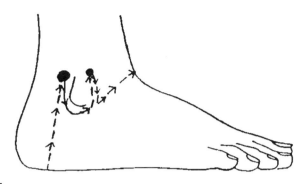

DIAGRAM 37
RIGHT FOOT
(Outer side)

BREAST AREA

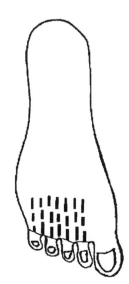

DIAGRAM 38
RIGHT FOOT
(Top)

BONES OF THE HAND

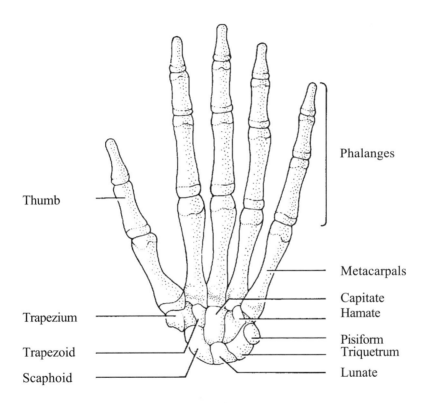

Phalanges

Thumb

Metacarpals

Capitate
Hamate

Trapezium

Pisiform
Triquetrum

Trapezoid

Scaphoid

Lunate

REFLEXOLOGY ROUTINE

LEFT FOOT

1.   DIAPHRAGM / SOLAR PLEXUS

Z 1 TO Z 5 AND Z 2/3

Gently push all the toes backwards with one hand. This will make the
diaphragm line more visible. While holding this position use thumb of free
hand to work along the diaphragm line from Z 1 to between Z 2 and Z 3 solar
plexus. Stop at this point turn thumb so tip is pointing towards the toes and
press three times. Then continue to work across the foot on diaphragm line to
Z 5. Then repeat the entire process.

2.   HEAD AND BRAIN

Z 1 TOE ONE

Work with the thumb from the base of the big toe (outside edge) up the outside,
over the top and down the inner side (in a horseshoe shape). Return to the start
point and repeat the movement. **Return** to the start point again, only this time
work from the base of the big toe underneath to the top. Continue this
movement until the base area of the big toe is treated (X 2). Now work on the
top of the toe in a similar way; only this time work from the **bottom of the nail** to
the bottom of the toe. Make sure to treat the whole area of the top of the toe X
2.

Areas of the Toe
Treatment of the upper part of the toe area is covering the whole face (nose,
mouth, jaws, gums, and teeth).

Treatment over the top and sides of the toe is covewring the brain, cranial
nerves, sides of the head and ears.

Treatment on the base of the toe sole is covering the back of the head including
the systems connected with it (bones, muscles, nerves, blood supply, brain
etc.).

DIAPHRAGM / SOLAR PLEXUS

DIAGRAM 1
LEFT FOOT
(Sole)

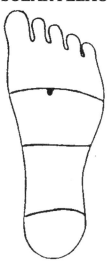

HEAD AND BRAIN

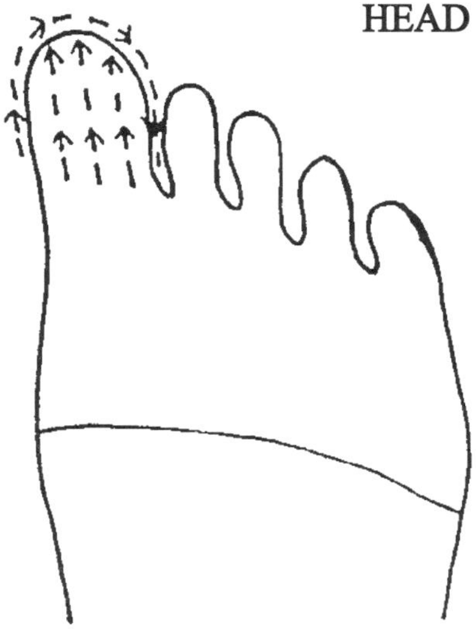

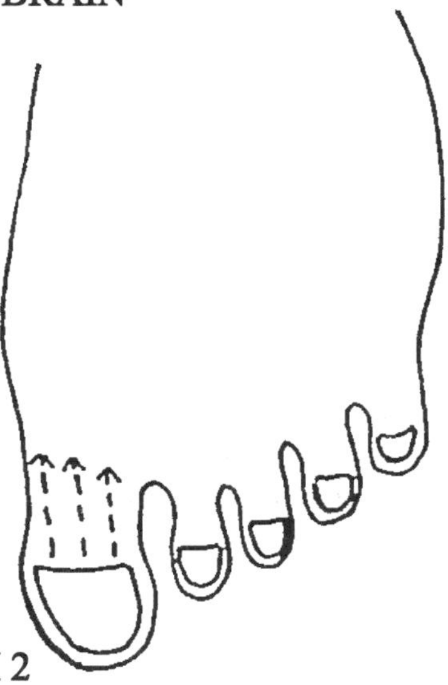

DIAGRAM 2
LEFT FOOT

3.   FRONT OF NECK/GENERAL NECK
Z 1 TOE ONE

Put index finger at the base of the big toe; on top of the foot. Work across this base line from the outside of the toe to the inside. Stop between toe 1 and toe 2. Then return to start point and repeat the movement X 2. Making a total of three movements.

Treatment of this area is covering all the structures of the neck/throat, thyroid, parathyroid, tonsils, epiglottis, vocal cords, eustachian tubes (reactions in the lymph tissue of the tonsils is found on the side of the big toe at its base next to Z 2). There is a very small point on the median line at the base of the great toe on the neck reflex that will sometimes react when the tonsil is energy starved.

4.   BACK OF NECK/GENERAL NECK
Z 1 TOE ONE

Work in a straight line across the base crease of the big toe (underneath). Start from outside edge. Work to inside (between toe 1 and toe 2). Return to start point and repeat X 2.

Treatment of this area is covering muscular and skeletal structures of the neck as well as all the points found in the front of the neck area.

Note. The base of the toe is very small therefore all the structures of the neck are to be found in both the front and back. However experience has proven that certain areas react more favourably on one side than the other.

FRONT OF NECK

DIAGRAM 3
LEFT FOOT
(Top)

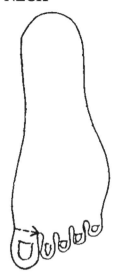

BACK OF NECK

DIAGRAM 4
LEFT FOOT
(Sole)

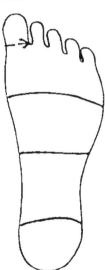

122

5.   OCCIPITAL

Z 1 TOE ONE

Use thumb to caterpillar walk up the base of the big toe close to the inside edge. Start the movement from the base crease line (neck area) and make 3 very small movements up towards the top of the toe. Stop and give 3 definite presses.

Note.   This movement is performed on the base of the toe not the inner side.

6.   EAR POINT / MASTOID PROCESS

Z 1 TOE ONE

Work up toe from occipital point 1 further movement to the mastoid process. Give 3 definite presses.

6A. TEMPLE

Work up from the mastoid area for two small points to just below the crown of the top of the toe. Give three definite presses.

OCCIPITAL

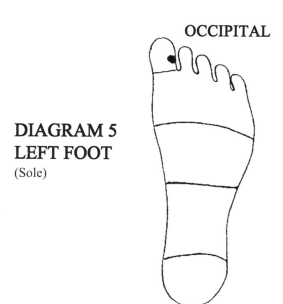

**DIAGRAM 5
LEFT FOOT**
(Sole)

EAR POINT - MASTOID PROCESS

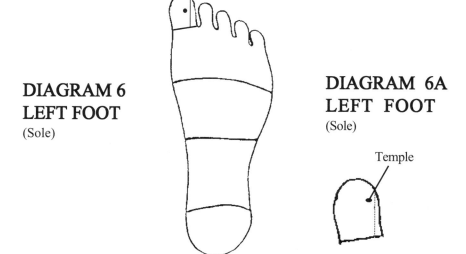

**DIAGRAM 6
LEFT FOOT**
(Sole)

**DIAGRAM 6A
LEFT FOOT**
(Sole)

Temple

124

7.   PITUITARY

Z 1 TOE ONE

Place thumb in centre of pad on the big toe pointing towards the top of the toe. Press X 3.

Note. When treating a client who suffers from Acne type skin or if there are any problems related to the endocrine system in general press and release X 3 again.

7A. PINEAL GLAND / HYPOTHALAMUS

Place the thumb on the pituitary gland, move one very small point up towards the top of the toe. Rock the thumb over onto its outer edge and give three pressure type circles (using the outer edge of the thumb). Without lifting the thumb, rock the thumb over onto its inside edge and give three pressure type circles using the inside edge of the thumb.

Note.   Neither set of pressure circles will be given directly on to the pituitary gland.

8.   SINUSES / CRANIAL NERVES

Z 2 TO Z 5. FOUR TOES

Work with the index finger from the base of the side of toe (between toe 1 and toe 2) up the side of toe two over the top and down the other side in a horseshoe shape. Repeat as on the big toe. Next work with the thumb from the base of the toe (underneath) to the top of the toe X 1. Work once more from the base of toe to the bulb, push the bulb up and gently backwards, as if trying to roll it over the top of the toe. Treat all toes 2 to 5

Note.   The area of the cranial nerves will be found on the sides of the toes.

Note.   Where sinus problems or headaches exist repeat the entire movement (No.8) twice

125

PITUITARY

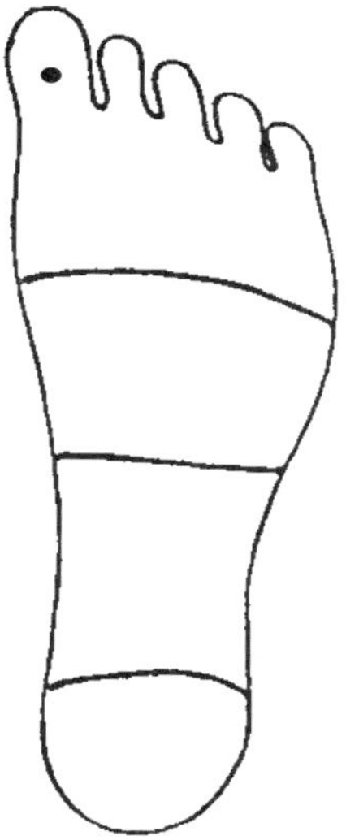

DIAGRAM 7
LEFT FOOT
(Sole)

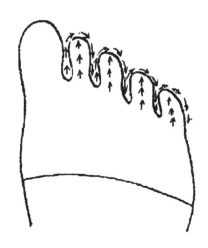

DIAGRAM 7A
LEFT FOOT
(Sole)

Pineal
Hypothalamus

SINUSES

DIAGRAM 8
LEFT FOOT
(Sole)

9.   TEETH

Z 1 TO Z 5. FIVE TOES

This time work on top of the toes. Start at the base of the nail and work down
to the bottom of each individual toe X 2. Do as many movements as are
necessary to cover the whole width of the toe from nail to base.

Note. All teeth are treated on the big toe in general
          Incisors and Canine teeth   toe 2
          Premolars   toe 3
          Molars   toe 4
          Wisdom   toe 5

10. LYMPHATICS OF HEAD / NECK

Z 1 TO Z 5 BETWEEN TOES

Very gently pinch webbing between toes.

Note. When treating webbing between Z 1 and Z 2 especially against the base
of the big toe a reaction may be noted. This area represents the tonsils helper.

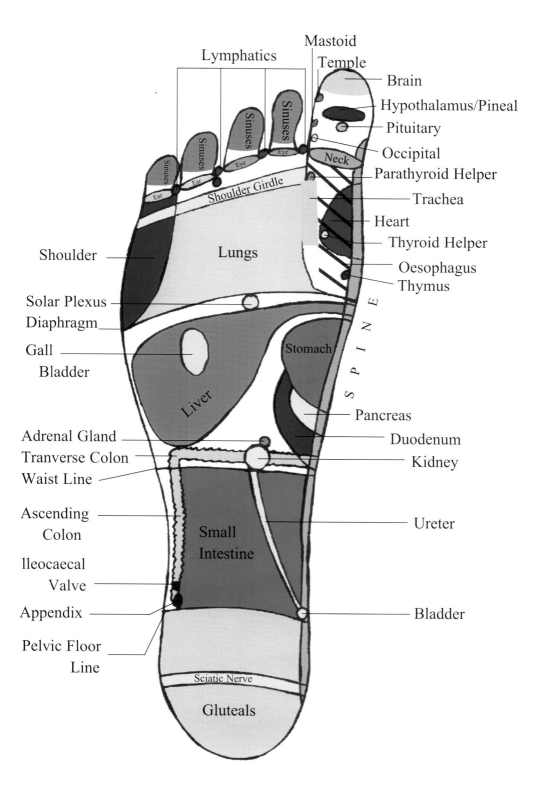

Lymphatics

Mastoid

Temple

Brain

Hypothalamus/Pineal

Pituitary

Occipital

Parathyroid Helper

Trachea

Heart

Thyroid Helper

Oesophagus

Thymus

Pancreas

Duodenum

Kidney

Ureter

Bladder

Shoulder

Solar Plexus

Diaphragm

Gall Bladder

Adrenal Gland

Tranverse Colon

Waist Line

Ascending Colon

lleocaecal Valve

Appendix

Pelvic Floor Line

Sinuses

Ear

Shoulder Girdle

Neck

Lungs

Stomach

SPINE

Liver

Small Intestine

Eye

Sciatic Nerve

Gluteals

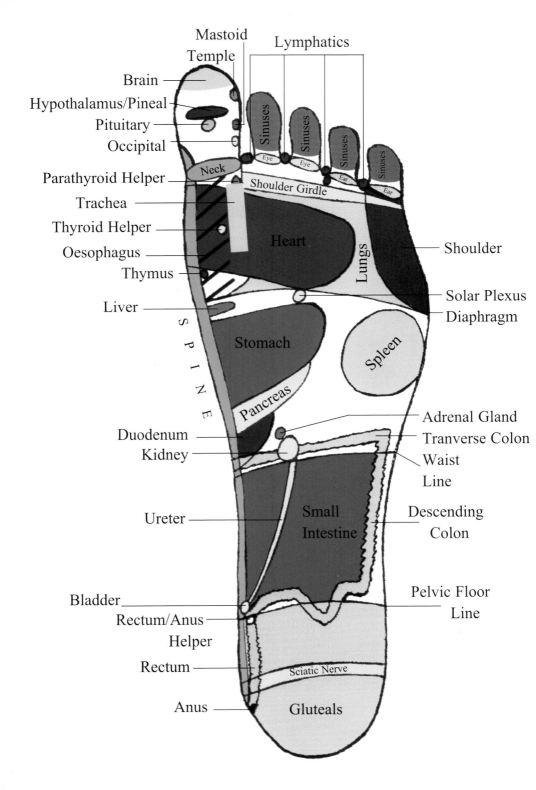

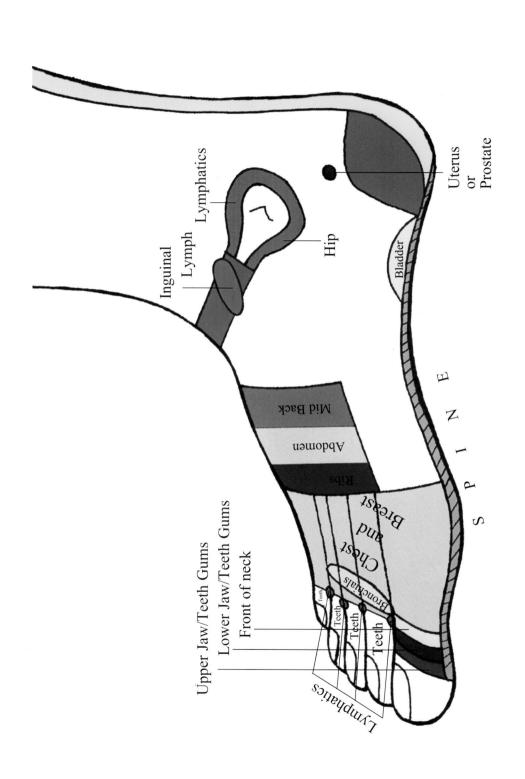

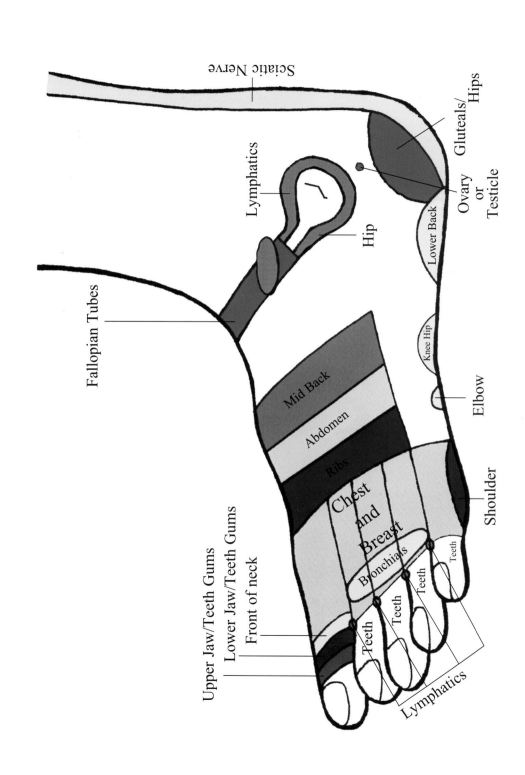

Sciatic Nerve

Gluteals/Hips

Lymphatics

Ovary or Testicle

Hip

Lower Back

Fallopian Tubes

Knee Hip

Mid Back

Elbow

Abdomen

Ribs

Shoulder

Chest and Breast

Upper Jaw/Teeth Gums

Lower Jaw/Teeth Gums

Front of neck

Bronchials

Teeth

Teeth

Teeth

Teeth

Teeth

Lymphatics

TEETH

**DIAGRAM 9
LEFT FOOT**
(Top)

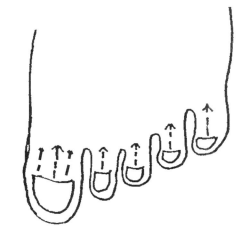

LYMPHATICS OF HEAD / NECK

**DIAGRAM 10
LEFT FOOT**
(Sole)

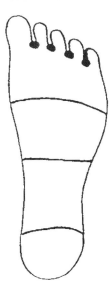

11. EYES / EARS

Z 2 TO Z 5 UNDER TOES

Bend toes back gently. With thumb of free hand work on top part of exposed pad along the top of the ridge at the base of the toes. Work from Z 2 to Z 5 X 2.

Note. eyes under Z 2/3 and **ears** under Z 4/5.

Remember that while working across this ridge pressure will in the main be in a downward movement with the medial aspect (inner side) of the thumb pressing against the base of the toes. It is also worth noting that sometimes there will be a reaction felt at the base of toe three (just above the metatarsophalangeal joint) when there is an energy blockage to the ear. This will always be confirmed when treating the ear area in Z 4 and Z 5.

12. EYE POINT

Z 2/3 UNDER TOES

Use thumb or index finger to press down firmly on the pad at the base of the toes (sole) between Z 2 and Z 3 (do not press into toes).

Note. This is a major helper reflex point to the eye, often reacting in people who normally wear contact lenses.

Note. A further reaction is sometimes felt at the base of toe 2 (just above the metatarsophalangeal joint) when there is an energy blockage to the eye. This will always be confirmed when treating the eye area between Z2 and Z3. The eye, like all the face, is also treated on the great toe.

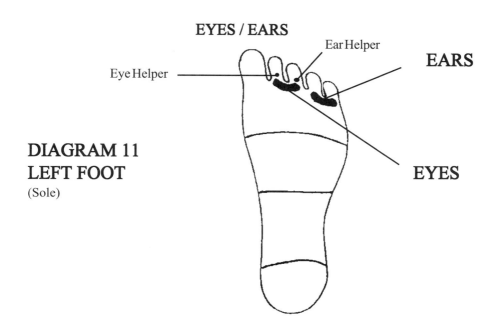

EYES / EARS

Ear Helper

Eye Helper

EARS

DIAGRAM 11
LEFT FOOT
(Sole)

EYES

EYE POINT - MAJOR HELPER

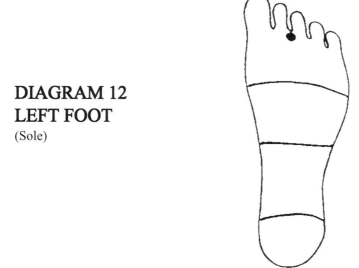

DIAGRAM 12
LEFT FOOT
(Sole)

13. EAR POINT

Z 4/5 UNDER TOES

Use thumb or index finger to press down firmly on the pad at the base of toes (sole) between Z 4 and Z 5 (Do not press into toes). This is a major reflex point for the ear often reacting in people who have had their ear syringed or in those who suffer with a wax problem.

Note. While this is a major reflex helper to the ear it should be remembered that the ear is treated also on the big toe and toe 3 with reflex points too small to be identified by all but the most experienced therapists. Middle ear problems often react on toe 3.

14. EUSTACHIAN TUBE

Z 3 / 4 UNDER TOES

Put the index finger of one hand at the base of the toes between Z 3 and Z 4 on the top of the foot. Put the thumb of the same hand on the sole at the base of the toes (on the pad) between Z 3 and Z 4. Push down firmly towards the heel while pinching together gently. This hold is on the fleshy area not on or between the toes.

Note. This is a helper reflex point for the eustachian tube (eustachian tube also treated on the big toe).

EAR POINT - MAJOR HELPER

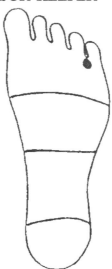

DIAGRAM 13
LEFT FOOT
(Sole)

EUSTACHIAN TUBE

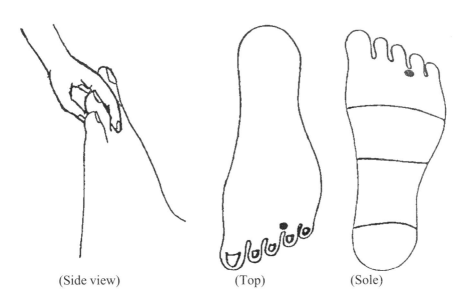

(Side view)   (Top)   (Sole)

DIAGRAM 14
LEFT FOOT

15. BALANCE

Z 4 TOE FOUR

Slide index finger down toe 4 on top from nail to base; then press into base X 2.

16. SHOULDER POINT / LYMPHATICS
Z 4/5 TOP OF FOOT AND SOLE

Use index finger to slide down from the base of the toes (top of foot) between toe 4 and toe 5 to just below the knuckle area (metatarsophalangeal joint). Put the thumb on the corresponding point on the sole area of the foot, press firmly X 2. **Hold the thumb and finger in the grip position, allow hand to fall to the side and work with seven circular movement while maintaining the grip.**

Note. Fingers and thumb should not slide over the flesh for this movement but should be held in position while the flesh is moved.

BALANCE

DIAGRAM 15
LEFT FOOT
(Top)

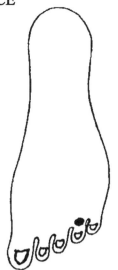

SHOULDER

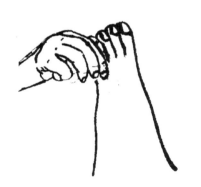

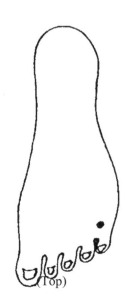

(Outer side)

(Top)

DIAGRAM 16
LEFT FOOT

17. THYROID / PARATHYROID / THYMUS / BRONCHI / TRACHEA
(general area helper)
(ZONAL)

Z 1 SOLE

Place the thumb on the diaphragm line at the outer edge of Z 1 toe 1. Begin caterpillar like walk towards Z 2 but stop between Z 1 and Z 2. Turn the thumb to point towards the toes and work up crease line to between big toe and toe 2. Return to start point and repeat entire movement.

17A. THYROID (ZONAL)

Z 1 SOLE

Lift the thumb and place it in the centre of the pad of the ball of the foot Z 1. Move one point up towards the base of the big toe and give three pressure circles.

THYROID / PARATHYROID / THYMUS / BRONCHI / TRACHEA (GENERAL AREA TREATMENT)

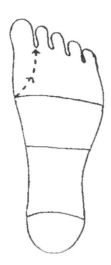

DIAGRAM 17
LEFT FOOT
(Sole)

THYROID

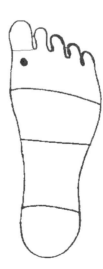

DIAGRAM 17A
LEFT FOOT
(Sole)

17B.   PARATHYROID (ZONAL)

Z 1 SOLE

Lift the thumb and place it in line with the thyroid on the edge of zone one (next to Z 2); move thumb one point up towards the base of the big toe and give three pressure circles.

17C.   THYMUS (ZONAL)

Z 1 SOLE

Lift the thumb and place it in line with the thyroid; move one tiny point down and one tiny point out towards the edge of the foot (as close to the edge of the foot as possible while still working on the sole). Give three pressure circles.

18. OESOPHAGUS / TRACHEA

Z 1 SOLE

Place the thumb on the diaphragm line at the edge of Z 1 (medial aspect of foot). Work from this point up to the base of the big toe. Return to diaphragm line and continue to work to base of toe until the entire pad has been treated in this way.

Note. Two thirds of this area represents the oesophagus (working from edge of foot towards Z 2) the other third represents the trachea. Two points up from the diaphragm line the trachea/bronchi (area one third closest to Z 2) enter the lungs. Also note that on Z 1 working up for 1 point from diaphragm lies the reflex area for a hiatus hernia. (See diagram opposite)

PARATHYROID

**DIAGRAM 17B
LEFT FOOT**
(Sole)

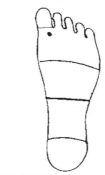

THYMUS

**DIAGRAM 17C
LEFT FOOT**
(Sole)

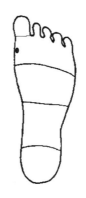

OESOPHAGUS / TRACHEA

Hiatus
hernia

**DIAGRAM 18
LEFT FOOT**
(Sole)

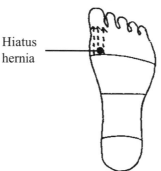

19. CHEST / LUNGS / SHOULDER
Z 2 TO Z 5 SOLE

Put thumb on diaphragm line directly under Z 2 (edge of Z 1). Work from diaphragm line to base of toes. Continue to work in this manner until the entire area from Z 2 to Z 5 has been treated. Repeat movement.

Note. When working from diaphragm line Z 5 to base of toe 5 reactions will give indications of shoulder reflex not lungs. Reactions occuring between Z 2 and Z 4 indicates lungs.

Note. Exercise caution in this area if a pace maker is fitted.

19A. SHOULDER GIRDLE / SCAPULA

On the sole of the foot just below the toes is a ridge prominence. One tiny point below this ridge Z 1 to Z 5 is the reflex point for the shoulder girdle, scapula and clavicle.

Note. This area is treated with number 19 and is thus not treated again unless a reaction is felt. Should a reaction be felt then this area should be treated separately as follows :- Work across the reflex from Z 1 to Z 5 X 2.

20. CHEST / LUNGS CONTINUED
Z 1 TO Z 5 TOP OF FOOT

This time work on top of the foot and use the index finger and not the thumb. Start at the base of the big toe and work with caterpillar movements down the foot towards the ankle, to a point corresponding to the diaphragm line. Treat all five zones in this manner. When the area has been treated return to the start point and repeat the process.

Note. This area is also treating the ribs and general musculature of the chest

CHEST / LUNGS

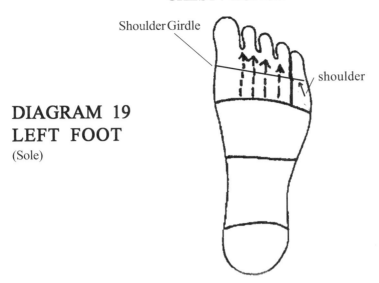

DIAGRAM 19
LEFT FOOT
(Sole)

Shoulder Girdle

shoulder

CHEST / LUNGS - CONTINUED

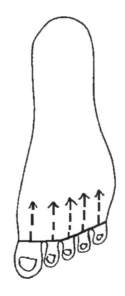

DIAGRAM 20
LEFT FOOT
(Top)

21. UPPER ABDOMEN
Z 1 TO Z 5 SOLE

Do not treat this area if a heart monitor/support device box is fitted within this area.

Put thumb on diaphragm line Z 1 as close to the edge of the foot as possible. Work across the foot from Z 1 to Z 5. Continue to work in this manner until the entire area between diaphragm line and waist line has been treated. Return to start point and repeat movement.

Note. Just above the waist line on Z 1 (see diagram) is found the reflex point for the Pyloric Sphincter

22. CARDIAC / HEART AREA (LEFT FOOT ONLY)
CHEST AREA

Do not treat area if pacemaker or heart monitor fitted.

Put the thumb just above the diaphragm line on Z 3 / Z4 pointing towards Z 1. Press and release X 2. Put the index finger on the top of the foot in area corresponding to thumb position on the sole. Press X 2 then work seven gentle massage pressure circles with the index finger. These pressure circles cover the area between Z 4 and Z 1. Remove the index finger. Use the thumb to give seven gentle massage circles on the sole of the foot. As with the index fingers these pressure circles should cover area from Z 4 to Z 1.

Important! Do not return to the cardiac area even if sensitivity is felt.

Note. The lesser heart reflex also passes into Z 1 on right foot (already treated).

UPPER ABDOMEN

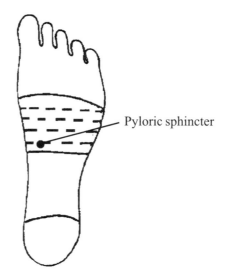

DIAGRAM 21
LEFT FOOT
(Sole)

Pyloric sphincter

CARDIAC / HEART AREA

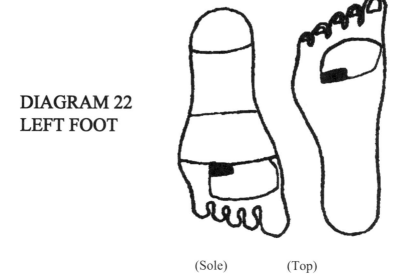

DIAGRAM 22
LEFT FOOT

(Sole)   (Top)

23. SPLEEN (LEFT FOOT ONLY)
Z 4 TO Z 5 SOLE

Place the thumb on Z 4 facing towards Z 5 below the diaphragm line. Work across Z 4 and Z 5 in three straight rows. On completion repeat this movement working this time from Z 5 to Z 4. If difficulties are being experienced working in opposite direction then work in one direction only (repeat movement)

Note. The main reflex point for the spleen will show up on Z 5

24. STOMACH / PANCREAS / DUODENUM
Z 1 TO Z 3 SOLE

Do not treat if heart monitor/support device box is fitted.

Place the thumb just below diaphragm line on the sole close to the median line (to the edge of the foot). By placing the thumb flat on the sole with the inner edge against the diaphragm line you will be in the correct place to commence. Work from Z 1 to Z 2 across the foot in three straight but slightly overlapping rows. On completion of the three rows repeat the movement in the opposite direction. If experiencing difficulty in changing hands or working in the opposite direction then return to start point and repeat the movement as before.

Line 1   Stomach
Line 2   Pancreas
Line 3   Pancreas / Duodenum

Exercise great care when dealing with a diabetic or a client who is suffering stomach ulcers (work very gently).

SPLEEN

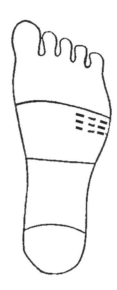

**DIAGRAM 23
LEFT FOOT**
(Sole)

STOMACH / PANCREAS / DUODENUM

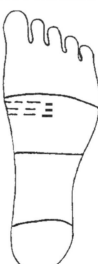

**DIAGRAM 24
LEFT FOOT**
(Sole)

25. LOWER ABDOMEN / SMALL INTESTINE
Z 1 TO Z 5 SOLE

Put thumb on waist line, work with caterpillar like movement from Z 1 to Z 5 until entire area between waist line and pelvic floor line has been treated. Repeat movement in opposite direction i.e. Z 5 to Z 1.

Important Note - Though some therapists work this area upwards (longitudinal) my experience has shown that the recipient has a tendency to feel sick. I have proven to my own satisfaction that to work across the foot gives better results.

25A LOWER BACK \ PELVIS \ SCIATIC
(general zonal helper area)
Z 1 TO Z 5

Put the thumb on the hard heel pad just below the pelvic floor line. Work with caterpillar like movements across the foot from Z 1 to Z 5. Treat entire heel pad area. When area has been treated in this direction then caterpillar walk upwards on each zone from base of heel to pelvic floor line (treat entire heel pad area). Do not repeat this movement

26. SCIATIC LINE
UP BACK OF LEG

Put one hand under leg, palm uppermost (against leg). Then with a slow, sliding type, push movement, work from ankle up to behind the knee; return to the start point and repeat X 2. Return to start point again, this time close heel of hand onto leg in a squeezing movement, work up leg to behind knee. Return to start point and repeat X 2.

LOWER ABDOMEN / PELVIS / SMALL INTESTINE

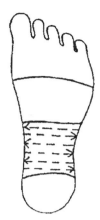

**DIAGRAM 25
LEFT FOOT**

SCIATIC LINE

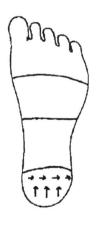

DIAGRAM 26

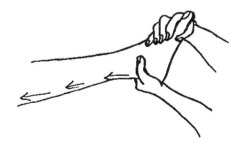

**DIAGRAM 25A
LEFT FOOT**

27. SCIATIC LINE - CONTINUED
BEHIND ANKLE - ACROSS SOLE

Put thumb of one hand (pointing down towards the sole) on the soft flesh area behind the ankle bone at its highest point. Work with caterpillar like movements down behind ankle bone then across the hard heel pad on the sole of the foot (change hands if necessary) and continue to work with this movement up behind the other ankle bone to its highest point. Return to start point and repeat movement X 2. (Total of three).

Note. On hard heel pad (sciatic line) between Z 3/4 there is likely to be a reaction when sciatic problems exist. Treat in usual manner with pressure circles.

28. SPINE
INNER EDGE OF FOOT

Use the thumb to work with caterpillar like movements down inner edge of foot (medial aspect) from just below nail area on big toe to the heel. Follow the curve of the foot (feeling for the bone). Repeat movement in opposite direction from heel to toe, then repeat entire movement. When a reaction is felt over a large area of the spine repeat the spinal walk up to a total of seven times depending on general reactions.

1   Cervical spine from base of toe nail to one point down from base of toe
2   Thoracic spine from two points down from the base of the toe crease to
        two points above waist line
3   Lumbar vertebrae from one point above the waist line to three points
        below waist line
4   Sacrum and Coccyx from four points down from waist line to the end
        of the spinal reflex point

Note. Due to the huge supply of nerves directly from the spinal cord to the body, treating the spine works not only on the skeletal and muscular structure of the area but gives a general treatment to all the organs/structures of the body.

SCIATIC LINE - CONTINUED

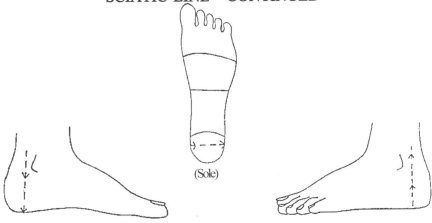

(Sole)

DIAGRAM 27
LEFT FOOT

SPINE

DIAGRAM 28
LEFT FOOT
(Sole & Medial View)

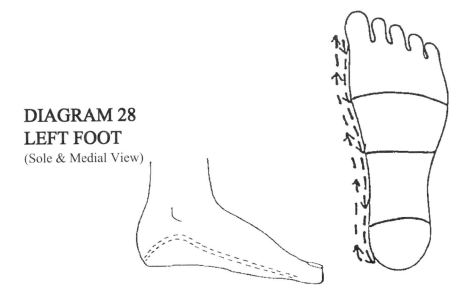

29. SHOULDER / ELBOW / KNEE /HIP / LOWER BACK
OUTER EDGE OF FOOT

Use the thumb to work with caterpillar like movement down outer edge of the foot from below nail area on little toe to the heel (first three walks are treating the shoulder reflex). Repeat movement in opposite direction then repeat the entire movement.

29A ELBOW HELPER (Treat if problem present)

Caterpillar walk down outer edge of foot for four points (2 points below the 5th metatarsophalangeal joint). Turn thumb and caterpillar walk on to the top of the foot for three points, then give three pressure circles.

29B KNEE HELPER (Treat if problem present)

Immediately the protrusion on the side of the foot is felt (base of the fifth metatarsal) caterpillar walk on to the top of the foot for five points. Give three pressure circles. When a knee problem exists and no sign of energy blockage is evident turn the thumb and work up towards the toes on a level with the elbow reflex. Press X 5

29C HIP HELPER (Treat if problem present)

Caterpillar walk from the end of the protrusion (end nearest heel) in a diagonal line to the base of the ankle. Change hands and caterpillar walk down from the base of the ankle in a straight line to the edge of the heel. Caterpillar walk up from the edge of the foot to the base of the ankle to fill in the gap in the triangle.

30. RECTUM / ANUS / LOWER PELVIS
Z 1 TO Z 5

Put thumb on outer edge of heel in line with ankle (pointing towards the floor with the fingers resting on the sole of the foot). Work with caterpillar movement around behind the heel to the corresponding point on the opposite side which is just one point below the bladder reflex. Stop and give three pressure circles on this reflex area of the rectum/anus. Return to start point and repeat the movement. **Note.** This movement is completed in a horseshoe shape, but it may be commenced from medial aspect (inner side of the foot) or the lateral aspect (outside of foot). Just remember to give three pressure circles on the rectum/anus helper point (inner side of foot)

SHOULDER / ELBOW / KNEE / HIP / LOWER BACK

DIAGRAM 29
LEFT FOOT
(Sole)

DIAGRAM 29C
LEFT FOOT

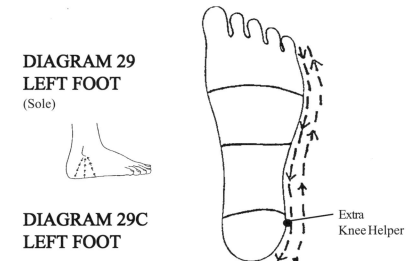

Extra
Knee Helper

RECTUM / ANUS / LOWER PELVIS

DIAGRAM 30
LEFT FOOT
(Sole)

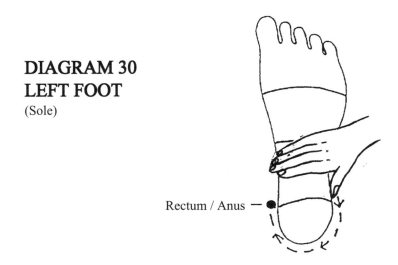

Rectum / Anus

31. KIDNEY / URETER TUBES

Place thumb to straddle the waist line between Z 2 and Z 3. Use left hand on right foot. With tip of thumb pointing towards toes press and release X 2. Remove thumb, replace thumb and press and release X 2 again. Swivel thumb around so that the tip of the thumb is pointing towards heel, work down the ureter tubes (Z 2) along the side of the tendon to the hard heel pad. Twist hand around, still using thumb, walk up the side of the foot (medial aspect) to centre of the bladder (between three and four points/walks up onto side of foot) press X 3 (bladder usually is a slightly puffy area on the inside of the foot). See number 32 for information on the bladder.

32. BLADDER

INNER SIDE OF FOOT

The bladder is usually visible as a slightly puffy area between three and four points/walks up onto the medial aspect of the foot proximal to the pelvic floor line (big toe side - see diagram) Place the thumb in the centre of the bladder area then work in points radiating outwards. (Use three small caterpillar like movements for 4 lines).

Do not work back up ureter tubes towards kidney as this may transfer any infection present in the bladder to the kidney. To treat in this way would work against the way nature has designed the system to work.

KIDNEY / URETER TUBES

DIAGRAM 31
LEFT FOOT

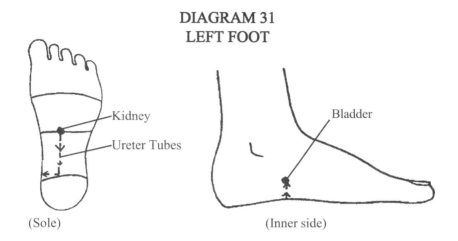

Kidney

Ureter Tubes

Bladder

(Sole)

(Inner side)

BLADDER

DIAGRAM 32
LEFT FOOT
(Inner side)

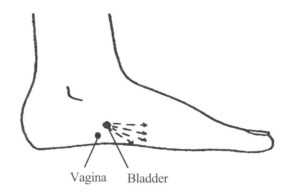

Vagina Bladder

33. ADRENALS

Z 1/2

Put one thumb on the kidney point pointing towards toes and bring second thumb to meet it (on the big toe side). This thumb should be pointing towards the heel. Now both thumbs should be pointing in opposite directions with nails almost parallel. Remove the thumb from the kidney point. With the remaining thumb on the adrenal gland press and release gently X 3. If client/patient suffers with acne type skin or there are any problems related to the endocrine sytem then press this area a further three times.

34. UTERUS / PROSTATE

BELOW INNER ANKLE

Place index finger on inner ankle bone.

Place third finger on tip of heel.

Bend second finger slightly, it will fall in line with the other fingers. When the point of importance has been located by middle finger, remove all three fingers and place the thumb on point where the middle finger rested. Press and release X3.

This location movement can be performed with the index finger on the heel and the third finger on the ankle bone, if this is found to be a more comfortable position for the therapist.

Note. If IUD is fitted work with great care and do not press directly on to the uterus area

ADRENALS

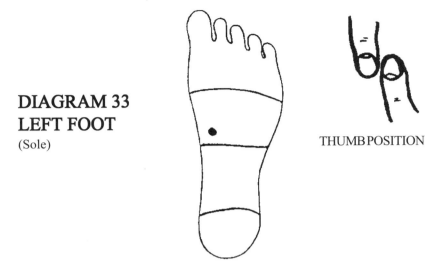

DIAGRAM 33
LEFT FOOT
(Sole)

THUMB POSITION

UTERUS / PROSTATE

DIAGRAM 34
LEFT FOOT
(Inner side)

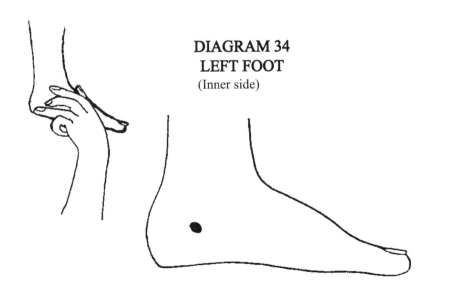

35. OVARIES / TESTES
BELOW OUTER ANKLE

Place index finger on outer ankle bone.

Place third finger on tip of heel.

Bend second finger slightly, it will fall in line with the other fingers. When the point of importance has been located by middle finger, remove all three fingers and place the thumb on point where the middle finger rested. Press and release X 3.

This movement can be performed with the index finger on the heel and the third finger on the ankle bone, if this is found to be a more comfortable position for the therapist.

Note. If the client suffers from Acne type skin or if there are any problems related to the endocrine system repeat the pressure X 3.

36. FALLOPIAN TUBES / VAS DEFERENS
TOP OF FOOT

Work with caterpillar like movement from outer ankle to inner ankle across crease line between foot and leg. Repeat this movement x 2.

OVARIES / TESTES

DIAGRAM 35
LEFT FOOT
(Outer side)

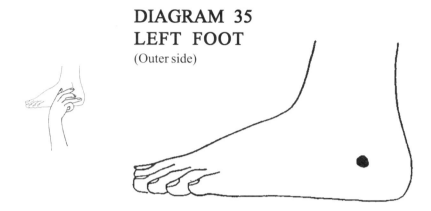

FALLOPIAN TUBES / VAS DEFERENS

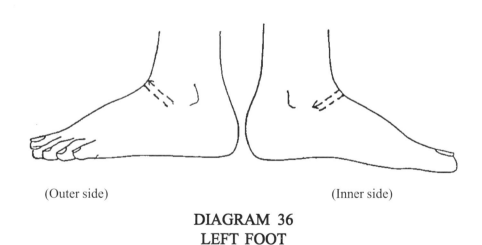

(Outer side)   (Inner side)

DIAGRAM 36
LEFT FOOT

37. LYMPHATIC / INGUINALS / PELVIC AREA

Place the thumb on the outer edge of the heel (see diagram) pointing upwards towards the leg.

Work up behind the ankle to an area one point higher than the ankle bone, press and release X 2. Then pull slide the thumb back to the bottom of the ankle and work around the base of the bone and up in front of the ankle bone (horseshoe shape) press X 2 one point higher than the ankle bone. Slide the thumb back to the base of the bone, turn the thumb and work across the leg-foot crease line to the other ankle. Change hands and repeat the whole process on the other ankle. Commence at the beginning again and repeat the movement on both ankles.
Note. This movement may be commenced on either ankle. Ensure both ankles are treated twice.

38. BREAST AREA
Z 2 TO Z 5 TOP OF FOOT

Use pad of index finger to work on the top of the foot in a gentle, slow, slide, press and release movement from the base of the toes to an area corresponding to the diaphragm line on the sole. Start movement at the base of toe 2. Work down Z 2, work back using a gentle pull and press movement. Work each zone 2 to 5 in this manner. This movement should be superficial.
Note. Return movement is almost like caterpillar walk in reverse.
It is important to remember that when working between the metatarsals the musculature of the chest are being treated as well as the more superficial breast. The ribs are represented by the metatarsals.

LYMPHATICS / INGUINALS / PELVIC AREA

**DIAGRAM 37
LEFT FOOT**
(Outer side)

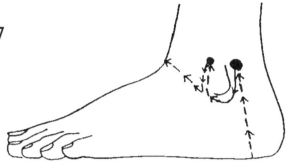

BREAST AREA

**DIAGRAM 38
LEFT FOOT**
(Top)

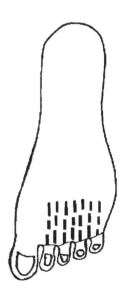

39. GENERAL ABDOMINAL / LOWER BACK AND CHEST BOOST

TOP OF BOTH FEET

Use both hands for this movement. Put one hand on each side of the edge of the foot just below the ankle; the fingers should be pointing into the edge of the foot, the thumbs should be on the sole. Slowly move fingers of both hands in a caterpillar like movement towards each other; work up the sides of the foot and onto the top. Treat the area between the ankle and base of toes. This may be repeated once or twice depending on the client's reactions.

39 A.   RETURN TO RIGHT FOOT AND REPEAT STEP 39.

40. COLON

SOLES OF BOTH FEET

Commence with the right foot. Place the thumb on the pelvic floor line in Z 4 / Z5 with tip pointing towards Z 1. Press X 4 (appendix and ileo caecal valve).

Turn the thumb around so tip points towards the toes and caterpillar walk up between Z 4/Z 5 to midway between waist and diaphragm line (ascending colon).

Turn thumb to point towards Z 1 (hepatic flexure) and caterpillar across to Z 1 (transverse colon). Change to left foot and continue to caterpillar walk to between Z 4 and Z 5 (continuing transverse colon).

Turn the thumb to point towards the heel (splenic flexure) and caterpillar walk towards the heel to a level with the pelvic floor line.

Turn thumb to point towards Z 1 and caterpillar walk to between Z 3 and Z 4.

Turn tip of thumb towards the heel and give three deep pressure circles.

Turn thumb towards Z 1 and caterpillar walk to Z 1 at the edge of the foot. Press X 1 (major reflex for rectum)

Turn thumb and caterpillar straight down (rectum) to edge of heel.

Press X 3 (anus point).

Return to start point and repeat the movement X 2 (a total of three times)

LOWER BACK / GENERAL ABDOMINAL
AND CHEST BOOST

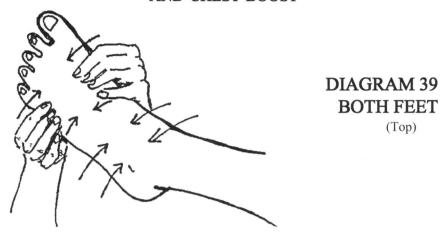

DIAGRAM 39
BOTH FEET
(Top)

COLON

DIAGRAM 40
BOTH FEET
(Sole)

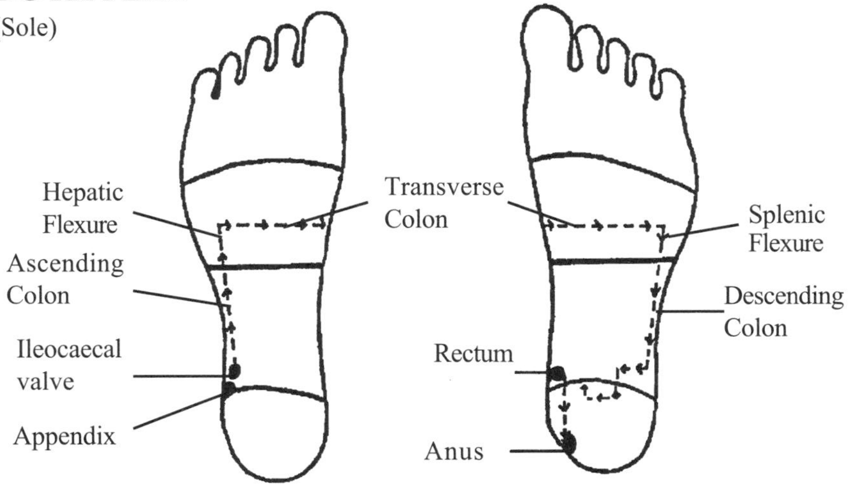

Hepatic Flexure

Ascending Colon

Ileocaecal valve

Appendix

Transverse Colon

Splenic Flexure

Descending Colon

Rectum

Anus

41. Return to treat any area that needs further treatment. (Both feet).

42. Work across diaphragm / solar plexus line. Treat solar plexus (both feet). Start with right foot.

43. Massage both feet starting on right foot.

44. Place your thumbs on solar plexus point of both feet and press gently three times. Some therapists like their clients to breath 'in' as they press on the solar plexus and 'out' as they release the pressure. (Be careful as this might cause the client to feel dizzy).

45. Leave client on couch or chair asking them to relax and not to move .

46. While the client is relaxing go and wash your hands.

47. Help the client off the couch /chair and assist them in dressing.

48. Make a further appointment if necessary.

49. Complete consultation/record card.

50. Wash your hands.

MEMORY JOGGER

1	x 3	Press	Diaphragm / Solar Plexus
2	x 3	Walks	Head / Brain
3	x 3	Walks	Front of neck
4	x 3	Walks	Back of neck
5	x 3	Press	Occipital
6	x 3	Press	Ear / Mastoid Process
6A	x 3	Press	Temple
7	x 3	Press	Pituitary
7A	x 3	Press	Pineal /Hypothalamus
8	x 4	Walks (2 x 2)	Sinuses/Cranial Nerves
9	x 2	Walks	Teeth
10	x 1	Pinch	Lymphatics of Head and Neck
11	x 2	Walks	Ears / Eyes
12	x 1	Pinch	Eye point
13	x 1	Press	Ear Point
14	x 1	Pinch / Press	Eustachian Tube
15	x 2	Press	Balance
16	x 2	Press x 7 Circles	Shoulder Point
17	x 2	Walks	Thyroid / Parathyroid / Thymus Area
17a	x 3	Circles	Thyroid
17b	x 3	Circles	Parathyroid
17c	x 3	Circles	Thymus
18	x 2	Walks	Oesphagus / Trachea
19	x 2	Walks	Chest Lungs - Sole of Foot
19A	x 2	Walks	Shoulder Girdle/Scapula
20	x 2	Walks	Chest Lungs - Top of Foot
21	x 2	Walks	Upper Abdomen
22	x 2	Press	Right Foot Only - Gall Bladder
23	x 2	Walks x 3 Rows	Right Foot Only - Liver
24	x 2	Walks x 3 Rows	Stomach / Pancreas / Duodenum
25	x 2	Walks	Lower abdomen / Pelvis / Small Intestine
25A	x 2	Walks	Lower back / Pelvis / Sciatic
26	x 2	Walks / squeezes	Sciatic Line
27	x 3	Walks	Sciatic Line - continued
28	x 4	Walks	Spine

29	x 2	Walks	Shoulder / Elbow / Hip / Knee / Lower Back
29A	x 3	Walks / Circles	Elbow Helper
29B	x 5	Walks x 3 Circles	Knee Helper
29C	x 3	Walks	Hip Helper
30	x 2	Walks x 3 Circles	Rectum / Anus / Lower Pelvis
31	x 4	Press x 1 Walk	Kidney / Ureter Tubes
32	x 3	Press / Walks	Bladder
33	x 3	Press	Adrenals
34	x 3	Press	Uterus / Prostate
35	x 3	Press	Ovaries / Testes
36	x 3	Walks	Fallopian Tubes / Vas-Deferens
37	x 4	Press x 4 Press	Lymphatics / Inguinals / Pelvic Area
38	x 2	Walks	Breast Area
39 /	x 2	Walks	Lymphatic / General Abdominal
			Chest Boost - Tops Both Feet
39A		Return to right foot	- Repeat 39
40	x 3	Walks	Colon - Both Feet
41		Return to treat areas as noted	
42	x 3	Press	Solar Plexus
43		Massage - Both Feet	
44	x 3	Press	Solar Plexus

REACTIONS
RELATED TO CONDITIONS

The following list (pages 165 - 179) is not meant to be diagnostic in any way. Neither is it intended to be used as a specific treatment routine. However, it may be used for treating symptomatically when a full treatment is not appropriate. I believe it is worthy of inclusion in my book, as it has been compiled from my own observations and faithful record keeping throughout my years of treating clients. In Reflexology, as in all other therapies, self education and re-education is very important. These findings might well encourage some therapists to compile and compare data for exchange, study and advancement of Reflexology.

During the normal reflexology routine reactions detected on all or the majority of the listed reflex points for a disorder or disease may denote the presence of the condition.

Not intended for treatment in a full reflexology routine

ACNE

The Pituitary
Thyroid / Parathyroid
The Liver
The Adrenals
The Kidneys
Diaphragm / Solar Plexus
The Ovaries in the Female / Testes, Prostate in the Male
The Lymphatic System

ALLERGIES

The Adrenals
The Ovaries and Uterus in Female / Testes, Prostate in Males
The Eyes
The Throat / Neck
The Liver
The Lymphatics
The Large and Small Intestines
The Solar Plexus
The Spleen

ANAEMIA

The Spine
The Spleen
The Liver

ANKLES

The Heart
The Adrenals
The Kidneys
The Sciatic
The Lymphatics

ARMPITS

Advise clients to have any abnormalities in this area checked by their medical practitioner.

The Shoulder
The Lymphatic System, Neck, Groin
The Solar Plexus

ARTHRITIS

The Solar Plexus
The Thyroid and Parathyroid
The Adrenals
The Kidneys
The Arm and Shoulder
The Spine
The Hip, Leg and Knee
The Head and Neck
The Lymphatic System

ASTHMA

The Solar Plexus
The Pituitary Gland
The Lungs
The Adrenals
The Large and Small Intestines
The Lymphatics
The Thyroid
The Spleen
The Head and Brain

BACK ACHE

The Solar Plexus
The Spine
The Shoulder, Arm, Hip and Leg

The Lymphatics
The Kidneys

BLADDER DISORDERS

The Solar Plexus
The Spleen
The Liver
The Adrenals
The Kidneys
The Bladder
The Lymphatics

BLOOD PRESSURE

The Solar Plexus
The Pituitary
The Thyroid and Parathyroid
The Heart
The Adrenals
The Kidneys

BREASTS

Provided a medical opinion has already been sought or the person is advised to see a medically qualified person, there is no reason why a complete Reflexology treatment cannot be given.

While we are aware that most breast abnormalities are harmless or if found not to be so, can be dealt with effectively if caught in time, the Reflexologist is not in a position to diagnose. He or she would be expected to behave in an ethical and professional manner in urging the sufferer to consult their doctor.

BREAST PROBLEMS BEFORE MENSTRUATION

The Pituitary
The Adrenals
The Kidneys
The Ovaries
The Lymphatics
The Breast
The Solar Plexus

BRONCHITIS

The Solar Plexus
The Lungs
The Adrenals
The Lymphatics

BURSITIS

The Adrenals
The Kidneys
The Shoulder
The Arm
The Hip
The Leg
The Lymphatics
The Bladder

CHOLESTEROL

The Thyroid
The Stomach
The Gall Bladder
The Liver
The Solar Plexus

COLD

It would be advisable for the therapist to wear a mask when treating this client.

COLITIS

The Adrenals
The Large and Small Intestines
The Lymphatic System
The Solar Plexus

CONSTIPATION

The Solar Plexus
The Stomach
The Pancreas
The Liver
The Gall Bladder
The Adrenals
The Large and Small Intestines
The Lymphatics

CRAMP (LEG)

The Thyroid and Parathyroid
The Hip, and Leg
The Sciatic Nerve
The Spine
The Lymphatics
The Solar Plexus

DIGESTION

The Liver
The Stomach
The Colon
The Solar Plexus
The Head
The Oesophagus
The Lymphatics

EAR DISORDERS

The Sinuses
The Ear. Eye and Balance Point
The Shoulder
The Spleen
The Solar Plexus
The Head/Brain

EYE DISORDERS

The Eye Reflexes
The Cervical Area on Spine
The Shoulder
The Sinuses
The Ears
The Solar Plexus
The Head/Brain

FEMALE DISORDERS (RELATED TO REPRODUCTIVE SYSTEM)

The Solar Plexus
The Pituitary
The Thyroid
The Spleen
The Liver
The Kidneys
The Adrenals
The Lymphatics
The Ovaries
The Uterus
The Fallopian Tubes

FLATULENCE (WIND)

The Stomach
The Liver
The Gall Bladder
The Large and Small Intestines
The Ileocaecal Valve
The Lymphatics
The Solar Plexus

FORGETFULNESS (STRESS RELATED)

The Solar Plexus
The Pituitary
The Brain
The Thyroid, Parathyroid and Thymus
The Adrenals
The Pancreas
The Spine
The Shoulder

GALL BLADDER

The Liver
The Gall Bladder
The Small and Large Intestines
The Kidneys
The Parathyroids
The Lymphatics
The Solar Plexus

GOUT

The Pituitary
The Spleen
The Adrenals
The Kidneys
The Intestines
The Solar Plexus
The Lymphatics

HAY FEVER

The Solar Plexus
The Pituitary
The Lungs
The Adrenals
The Spleen

HEADACHE

The Solar Plexus
The Brain
The Sinuses
The Ear
The Eye
The Stomach
The Pancreas
The Spine
The Shoulder

HEART DISORDERS

All heart conditions should be checked by a medically qualified practitioner.

INDIGESTION

The Liver
The Gall Bladder
The Stomach
The Solar Plexus
The Small Intestine
The Large Intestine (colon)

INFERTILITY (IN FEMALES)

The Solar Plexus
The Pituitary
The Thyroid
The Adrenals
The Ovaries
The Uterus
The Fallopian Tubes

IMPOTENCE AND INFERTILITY (IN MALES)

The Solar Plexus
The Pituitary
The Brain
The Thyroid and Parathyroid
The Testes
The Prostate
The Spleen
The Lymphatics

INSOMNIA

The Solar Plexus
The Brain
The Thyroid and Parathyroid
The Spine
The Shoulder
The Kidneys
The Bladder
The Lymphatics

KIDNEY DISORDERS

All kidney disorders should be diagnosed by a medically qualified practitioner.

The Pituitary
The Thyroid and Parathyroid
The Spleen
The Adrenals
The Kidneys and Ureter
The Bladder and Urethra
The Lymphatics

LIVER DISORDERS

All liver disorders should be diagnosed by a medically qualified practitioner.

The Thyroid and Parathyroid
The Liver
The Gall Bladder
The Spleen
The Kidneys
The Lymphatics

LUNG DISORDERS

Conditions of the lung, like all major organs, need to be investigated by a medically qualified practitioner.

The Solar Plexus and Diaphragm
The Lungs
The Adrenals
The Lymphatics

MENOPAUSE

The Solar Plexus
The Pituitary
The Thyroid and Parathyroid
The Ovaries
The Uterus
The Brain
The Lymphatics
The Adrenals

MENSTRUAL (PREMENSTRUAL TENSION)

The Pituitary
The Brain
The Thyroid and Parathyroid
The Adrenals
The Kidneys
The Ovaries
The Uterus
The Spine
The Solar Plexus

MIGRAINE

The Solar Plexus
The Brain
The Pituitary
The Heart
The Adrenals
The Kidneys
The Large and Small Intestines
The Sinuses
The Spine and Shoulder

NAUSEA

The Solar Plexus
The Brain
The Stomach
The Ear Reflex
The Balance Point
The Intestines (Large and Small)
The Adrenals

SCIATICA

The Sciatic
The Intestines (Large and Small)
The Spine
The Hip, Thigh and Leg
The Adrenals
The Sciatic Nerve
The Solar Plexus

SINUSITIS

The Pituitary
The Sinuses
The Intestines (Large and Small)
The Adrenals
The Lymphatic System
The Spleen

SKIN DISORDERS

The Solar Plexus
The Pituitary
The Thyroid
The Parathyroid
The Thymus
The Adrenals
The Liver
The Kidneys
The Gonads (Ovaries or Testes)
The Lymphatic System

STRESS

The Solar Plexus
The Pituitary
The Thyroid and Parathyroid
The Lungs
The Kidneys
The Adrenals
The Spine
The Shoulder, Hip, Leg
The Lymphatics

ULCERS (DIGESTIVE)

The Solar Plexus
The Stomach
The Intestines (Large and Small)
The Adrenals
The Liver
The Lymphatics

VARICOSE VEINS

The Heart
The Adrenals
The Hip and Leg
The Solar Plexus
The Intestines (Large and Small)
The Lymphatics

REVISION QUESTIONS

1   Who brought Reflexology to America?

2   Name the American woman who specialized in Reflexology.

3   How do the reflex points of Reflexology differ from the reflex points of the nervous system?

5   In Reflexology what is meant by reflex points?

6   Where are the Transverse Lines found?

7   What are the Longitudinal Zones?

8   What are the Crystals?

9   There are many reasons why a treatment may not be performed or when caution is needed. List not less than twelve.

10 Would you treat an Epileptic?

11 Are there any special precautions when treating a Diabetic?

12 What might happen if you overtreated a client?

13 Is it within the powers of a Reflexologist to refer people to their own doctor?

14 Give a list of Do Not's in Reflexology.

15 List seven rules of personal hygiene.

16 Name a contagious condition that affects the feet.

17 What should you do with the foot bowl after use?

18 With what should you cover the knee and foot rest?

19 Why is the comfort of both therapist and client important?

20   How should the client be kept warm?

21   While performing the initial foot examination what is the therapist looking for or observing on the feet?

22   Why is it important for the client to see the therapist's face?

23   Why is it not advisable to use oil, cream or talc in Reflexology?

24   If a Therapist thinks it is necessary to treat with an oil, cream or talc, then at what stage in the treatment can these products be used?

25   What homecare advice would you give to a client with excessively sweaty feet?

26   How much time would you allow for a first visit?

27   What sort of situation would dictate that the treatment should be given for 5/10 minutes instead of 40/45?

28   How does the treatment of a child differ from the treatment of an adult?

29   How often would you give a Reflexology treatment over the space of eight days?

30   What action does the therapist take when a crystal or sensitivity is felt?

31   Name the first area to be treated in the Reflexology Routine.

32   In what Zone does the head and brain lie?

33   Where would you massage for the pituitary?

34   Over what area on the foot is the spine treated?

35   In the 'Reflexology Routine' what organ/gland would you be working on between Z 1 to Z 5 between waist and pelvic floor line?

36   According to the routine in this book which would you treat first, the kidney or the bladder?

37   Define 'Contra Indicated'.

38   What sort of reaction might a client display during treatment?

39   Might a client suffer any reactions between visits to the therapist and if so what type of reactions might be expected?

40   Why is a consultation card necessary?

Answers to all these questions are found in the text.

SOME COMMON QUESTIONS ANSWERED

SOME COMMON QUESTIONS ANSWERED

Q   Are all Aromatherapists qualified Reflexologists?

A   No. Some Aromatherapists will have undertaken a separate course to qualify them in the field of Reflexology.

Q   I have been told that Reflexology is part of Aromatherapy. Is this true?

A   No! Some Aromatherapists do press on some Reflexology points in order to help them choose an oil for their Aromatherapy treatment; but this cannot be classified as Reflexology. However fortunately this is becoming a practice less often performed by the well qualified Aromatherapist.

Q   Are all Beauty Therapists Reflexologists?

A   No. Beauty Therapists who hold qualifications to undertake face and body treatments will have studied anatomy, physiology and massage. However, this does not qualify them as Reflexologists.

Q   Does the Reflexologist have to be insured?

A   All professional people should be insured.

Q   How can a Therapist get insurance to practice?

A   Therapists gaining their training through a recognised establishment will be given details of professional bodies/societies for membership and insurance.

Q   Where can I get information about courses?

A   By writing to one of the organisations listed on page 221, enclosing a stamped addressed envelope for your reply.

Q   If I experience problems finding local training at times to suit me how do I get help?

A   The author will help where possible in advising on seminars, lectures and open learning facilities run by her own organisation, Renbardou Training, but she is unable to enter into any other correspondence. (addresses can be found at the back of the book).

TEACHER TELL ME WHY AND WHEN.
I MIGHT HAVE TO ANSWER THESE QUESTIONS WHEN I AM ALONE

1.   **What is Reflexology ?**

The science that deals with the principle that there are reflex points on the hands and feet which correspond to all parts of the body's glands, organs and structures.

2.   **What are the benefits ?**

We have four main areas to look at :

1. To increase blood and lymph flow
2. To relieve stress and tension
3. To promote the unblocking of nerve impulses
4. To help the body maintain a state of balance

3.   **What does a cheese smell to the feet indicate ?**

The body is congested with waste and toxins (often constipated)

4.   **What does an Acetone smell indicate to the therapist ?**

This smell will suggest a possible urinary disorder not necessarily serious. It is sometimes evident in the diabetic

5.   **How much pressure do I use ?**

1. Depends on the type of foot being treated
2. Depends on the sensitivity of the client being treated
3. A heavy foot would need deep pressure
4. A slim, delicate foot would need a light pressure
5. A sick or frail person would need a light pressure
6. A child would need light pressure
7. A good guide is to observe the client's face
8. Ask for feedback

6. How many treatments ?

In this stressed world of ours ideally the therapist would like to recommend six to eight treatments. However I believe one treatment not only to be beneficial but financially realistic, especially when not dealing with a specific problem. The number of treatments and duration of each will depend on a number of factors.

7. Does the chronic condition and the acute condition react to the same number of treatments ?

No. The chronic condition will usually need more treatments before there are noticeable signs of improvement. The acute condition may require less than eight treatments while the chronic condition may require many more than eight

8. How many treatments should I give in order to establish the effectiveness of Reflexology ?

This is a difficult question to answer. However as a general guide it is best not to continue treatment after the third or fourth treatment if the client is unable to report any changes

9. How often do I treat ?

This very much depends on the client's condition and financial situation but once a week is ideal for most people as the reactions to treatment do not always show immediately but can take up to three or four days in some cases.
As a general guide the more sick the patient / client the more realistic is a weekly treatment. Should the reactions be very strong then the recipient of the treatment can be made to feel worse, giving them a greater burden to carry.

10. Are there any circumstances when I would treat more often then once per week ?

Yes. There are conditions that would benefit from a treatment more often then once a week but do assess your client very carefully.
A very fit client who suffers a sprain / strain could benefit from two or even more treatments in the space of one week.

An otherwise fit/healthy client who is suffering from P.M.S and / or pain can benefit from a twice weekly treatment but proceed with caution as P.M.S may show signs of getting worse before it gets better (the healing crisis). The client would always be advised of this possible reaction (these clients have always been amongst my most successful).

11.   Does Reflexology hurt ?

No. Reflexology should not hurt but some areas on the foot may feel tender or different.

12.   What does it mean if the client complains to the therapist of a bruising dull pain on the area being treated ?

This reaction seems to be experienced by those with more chronic conditions. However the therapist should very quickly establish that there is no injury to the foot in that area.

13.   What does it mean if the client complains of a very sharp pain, a sticking pain or a cutting pain in the area being treated ?

This type of reaction tends to be felt by those suffering with an acute condition but as always, the therapist would ensure that there was no injury to the foot

14.   What do I do if the client reaction is :

1. Hands perspiring

Continue the treatment but reduce your pressure

Cause : Reflex zone tends to be reactive at this time showing a stronger than normal reaction to treatment

2. All over perspiration

Stop the treatment. Hold the foot / hand for a little while then continue to treat but reduce the depth of pressure and give no pressure circles

Cause : A very strong reaction to treatment

3. A feeling of being very cold, especially in the limbs

Stop and cover client with an extra blanket or towel making sure that he / she is warm. Stroke the foot / hand gently for a few minutes. Return to Reflexology but this time make sure that the pressure is very gentle . Instead of the normal routine clear all zones, treat the solar plexus, the kidney, ureters and bladder, then treat the colon. Follow this with treatment of the solar plexus and a full foot / hand massage.

Cause : A very strong reaction to the treatment

15.   What are your views on treating cancer patients ?

Terminally ill patients will benefit from a specific treatment i.e. Diaphragm, solar plexus, zone walk, (sole and top) head, brain, spine, shoulder, hip, knee, gluteals, solar plexus and final massage.

Cancer patients will benefit from the above routine for the first treatment session. Therafter a normal treatment will encourage healing and well being. Pressure used should be lighter than normal.

Chemotherapy patients will benefit from a full reflexology treatment one or two days prior to their treatment and a zone walk as soon as possible after the chemotherapy (same day preferably)

16.   Would you treat a person with a fever ?

No. I do not as a rule. A fever might suggest a contagious condition. It may also put an extra burden on the healing process with which the body could not cope. However in recurrent fever with no apparent medical cause (especially in children) to treat the pituitary gland X 4 in the first hour followed by endocrine treatment has been known to produce good results. Allow two hours to elapse before returning to treatment

17.   What can you tell me about a corn on the foot ?

Corns are patches of hard skin which become dense in the centre. They can grow inwards right to the bone and can cause intense pain. Corns are found most frequently on toes 1, 3 and 4 and appear as a result of pressure from footwear. This protective shield will indicate to the therapist a possible reflex disturbance in the area due to the depth of inward growth.

18.   What can you tell me about a build up of hard skin ?

The foot forms hard skin to protect it from rough surfaces. This can be a ridge on the sole of a shoe, walking around bare foot or the natural posture and stance of a particular person. Hard skin that is flexible poses little threat to reflex disturbances but the thick, horny, inflexible skin often found on the heel, ball of the foot and the edge of the big toe, can indicate energy blockages.

19.   Can you remind me about the necessity for the consultation card.

1. To establish there are no contra indications to the treatment

2. To assess the client's physical and mental state

3. To show a genuine interest

4. To ensure that our therapy is holistic

5. To ensure that we give the best possible treatment for each client

6. To establish that Reflexology is the most suitable treatment

7. To refer client to a therapist with the appropriate skills or to a medically qualified practitioner.

20.   Why are we advised not to encourage general conversation during treatment but to always remember our listening skills and to deal with the client's needs?

Talking takes energy. Conversation about people puts the visual imagination to work, altering brain wave rhythms in the process. Thoughts are coloured by emotions and this in turn influences brain waves, dividing the brain's reflex action. Conversation may interfere with blood circulation since thoughts and emotions cause vascular changes, dilating or contracting blood vessels and altering normal rhythms of contraction and expansion. If conversation is related to the present the client/patient can focus on the sensations being felt at that moment. However the therapist must never loose sight of the fact that one of his/her greatest assets will be listening skills. Clients will sometimes like to talk about their lives. The therapist must not be judgemental though it is possible to perhaps suggest a different approach to the problem. The client's new approach to life may then help the body to function in a state of balance.

21. When the client asks, 'What exactly are you treating' ?

The Reflexologist treats the whole person through stimulating the nerve endings, the energy channels and vascular flow to the various organs and structures of the body which are reflected in miniature on the feet and hands.

22. Reflexology balances and revitalizes. What do you mean ?

Illness, stress, tension and fatigue can each have the effect of causing body disharmony (imbalance). Energy is wasted fighting the problem or struggling mentally with negative attitudes. Reflexology encourages the body's own energy flow and as the body and mind regain their balance they can work more efficiently.

23. If the bladder reflex was not just a puffy area on the side of the foot but stretches almost onto the sole.

Though there are a number of reasons it could in some cases indicate a full bladder or even a prolapsed bladder. A professional therapist would not make the latter statement to a client/patient.

24. An alcoholic asked me for help. Is there any point in treating ?

Yes indeed ! Do say that you will help but that it will be a joint involvement in the result. Do not treat the client whilst he / she is in a state of alcohol abuse / drunk. It is possible to encourage the client to gradually reduce their intake. In all cases I have treated I have found severe reactions on the entire endocrine system and I have given more treatment to the sensitive areas, but always in conjunction with a complete treatment. Over the course of the years I have successfully treated three alcoholics who, once the course of Reflexology had started, had no other form of treatment (various therapies had been tried previously).

25. The client is feeling unwell but no sensitivity is found during treatment. Why ?

Possible causes for lack of reactions:

1. The pressure is too light for the size / bulk of foot

2. Medication has in some way anaesthetised the reflexes

3. The client has a high pain threshold

4. There is a lot of congestion in the feet that needs clearing prior first

26.   When you say press, how long does the therapist press for ?

The therapist should count "one, two" distinctly (but not out loud) during the hold for each press

27.   What are the likely results of working for too long in any one session ?

To work for too long or indeed too deeply leads to the possibility of over stimulation, which can cause excessive elimination and discomfort. This in turn, can make the client feel that Reflexology is too unpleasant for them.

28.   What are the likely results of a treatment that is too short ?

In this case the body is not provided with sufficient stimulus to mobilise its own healing powers

29.   What is the energy ? Where does it come from ?

Chinese believe the whole functioning of the body and mind depends on the normal flow of energies which they call life force or chi, pronounced 'Chee', (in modern translation/interpretation sometimes called Qi pronounced 'K I').
Chi is a universal energy which pervades everything. We can neither see nor feel it, in much the same way as we cannot see nor feel Radio Waves or Ultra Violet

The energy in the body comes from the air we breathe and the food we eat. (There is no doubt that when we eat nutritionally rich food we are also taking in energy). Strong energy protects the body, acting as a defence system. The language of western medicine refers to this as a high resistance. If the chi is weak then the resistance is lowered which can result in illness of body or mind. Whether we think in terms of immune response or of chi, once illness has set in our inner resistance is of great importance in determining how easily therapist and the Reflexologist, through using their various methodologies are each aiming to strengthen and balance the energy flow. Reflex points are energy junctions that respond to pressure.

30. Why do books and charts differ in relation to reflex and zonal areas?

The body's organs and structures are always more or less in the same place but obviously muscle tone, age changes and heredity influences do have a bearing. All reflexologists agree with this statement. They further agree that no part of the body has its own precise compartment, all parts are forced to dwell in shared accommodation with there neighbours, muscles, blood vessels, nerves, and even other organs. A simple analogy could be packing a drawer in your bedroom or your suitcase to go on holiday, there is space for everything and everything has a space. However in Reflexology the therapist is packing the contents of the entire wardrobe into the bedroom drawer or holiday suitcase. In other words when the therapist is reflecting the entire body onto the feet each point of reflexion has to be very small, in some cases even minute. Therefore experience has taught that to support some of the reflexion points with helper areas that are either system or zonal linked will improve the overall value of the Reflexology treatment.

The reason why there tends to be some slight differences in reflex or zonal points is simple. It depends on whether the author includes all or most reflex points and helper areas or works only with some of the points that they consider important in order to gain the desired effect. For example some writers point out the inner ear only, whereas I put in all the ear treatment points and helper areas. What the student/therapist needs to be sure of is that the anatomical mapping and or the zonal mapping is being adhered to by the writer and that the originator of the text or chart has the knowledge and experience to produce material.

One example of anatomical mis-mapping in reflexology is, for example, the stomach being placed in the chest area above the diaphragm line. Another and more obvious one is when the breasts/mammary glands are placed on the chart below the waist line. It should be noted that a number of text books will use a combination of reflex and zonal points to gain the best response. Therapists who have worked for many years will always write books or publish charts based on their own clinical findings and documented notes, but there will to me always be a relationship in the writings. There are writers who have remained faithful to the original ideas and have not done independent studies or progressed on.

There are one or two books available that do differ quite considerably from the accepted norm. These books, are in my opinion, totally unsuitable for the student professional therapist, in that they bear little or no relationship to anatomical mapping or zonal relationships. Only the writings of the experienced therapist will be of value to the student of Reflexology. The qualified therapist will have the knowledge to be selective.

31. Should I treat during Pregnancy

During the first three months of pregnancy only the most experienced qualified therapist should treat. Thereafter only women with a good medical history may be treated by the less experienced therapist. A general routine omitting extra treatment on specific endocrine glands and the liver should maintain health throughout pregnancy.

Reflexology is known to relieve morning sickness and back aches well as boosting energy levels.

During labour Reflexology has many recorded benefits especially for relaxation and pain relief.

32. Can you give us a little more information about treating children ?

Children can respond very well to Reflexology treatment. The therapist should bear in mind that the child can have similar reactions to the therapy as would an adult, so treatment pressure, pace and duration would be judged accordingly.

The small child with little or no verbal communication skills will sometimes respond to sensitive reflexes by pulling the foot away and/or fidgeting, or even by clinging tightly to the parent or guardian.

The slightly older child (four - six years of age) is often chatty and usually happy to be told exactly what is happening; they are, in most cases, very accurate in their verbal response to a sensitive reflex.

The child of eight or nine years upwards requires that the therapist be particularly observant in noting changes in expression. At this age conditioning has often already taken place in relation to standards of acceptability with regard to complaining about levels of discomfort/hurt (the child might feel he/ she ought not to). Always ask for feedback, pleasant or otherwise.

The younger teenager will often be more relaxed in the absence of a parent or guardian. While I am not suggesting that the latter be precluded from the treatment area I have found that experience and intuition play a part in the therapist's decision to ask the parent/guardian for a little time alone with the child. This may of course be difficult or pose its own problems for example with opposite sexes or a first time visitor. I have found that some young people will not discuss problems in the presence of an accompanying adult, even problems such as school or peer bullying (at times the root cause of the problem).

The majority of children/teenagers are model patients/clients and love the attention of the one to one. In most cases they will confide in the therapist (don't worry, it may not happen on the first visit). The therapist should never dismiss anyone's fears let alone those of the child. All fears are real and never trivial to the one expressing them. Verbal reassurance coupled with a treatment can often work wonders.

In the above section I have chosen to mention those children who suffer no obvious handicaps but I do feel that a special mention is due to all those parents and the children who suffer a disability of any form. I have experienced the privilege of working with some such children and in all cases have been rewarded with a positive response (no matter how small). My successes have been as varied as with almost any other group :- from bowel regularity and improving sleep patterns to relaxation.

A special child case study
Robert, who throughout his eight years of life in total silence had not given even one recorded smile. Not only was Robert deaf, he had the mental age of a four year old and the obvious physical disability of having only one arm. I was asked by a friend to give Robert's mother a treatment as a birthday treat. She told me about Robert and asked if I could meet with him, though I did not normally make house calls I decided to make an exception and went off to meet Robert at 3.30 the next day.

I sat in the room close to the little boy for about a half hour before attempting to touch him. For most of the time he sat motionless, dwarfed by the huge armchair into which he had run and jumped upon my arrival. Though I knew Robert could not hear me I did make attempts to communicate with him using my eyes and lips and the various toys that lay around the room.

Eventually I held his feet and stroked one leg whilst observing the expressionless eyes. Robert's mother removed one of his shoes and I removed the other. I gave a few gentle effleurage movements to both feet followed by zonal clearing. I then treated: Solar plexus, head and brain, spine, eyes, ears,

194

eustachian tubes and completed the treatment with more effleurage of the feet. The treatment lasted in total about ten minutes. A week later I visited the family again Robert took up his position in the armchair and I repeated the exact process of the previous week. The only difference was that on this occasion I also massaged his hand. He squeezed my hand on two occasions when I had stopped the effleurage. This encouraged me to repeat both the foot and hand massage as it was my impression that he was enjoying the treatment.

The process was repeated in week three. This time Robert began squeezing my hand very tightly. When I had completed the treatment I playfully shook his hand with my left hand and still with a playful fashion rubbed the top of his head with my right hand. Robert moved in an effort to free himself from both my hands. While this was happening I was jerked into reality as his mother yelled out from behind me, 'He is smiling, he is smiling !' Well Robert was not the only one in the room smiling after we realised what he was doing. Although Robert tended to ration his smiles from then on, he would actually always give a big smile in response to having his hands effleuraged. He also learned to undo and remove his shoes and socks and make it very obvious that he wanted his feet treated. The respondent was usually treated to a beautiful smile. There are many children who may benefit from your care and efforts. I cannot tell you the joy of a response even if all are not as dramatic as Robert's.

The professional can pass on expert advice on how and when to perform movements that would be beneficial to a child (or adult), either between visits to the therapist or as an alternative to professional treatments.

FINALLY

No person or book can teach you what you will gain from experience and consolidation. A minimum of one year should be given over to laying the foundations after you qualify. The **International Federation of Reflexologists** have a Help Line for its members and local support group are present all over the UK. The I.F.R. now offer a number of courses in ungrading your knowledge. All these courses are supervised by top specialists and are advertised in the quarterly membership magazine, 'Stepping Out'.

Enjoy studying

Renée

ANATOMY & PHYSIOLOGY DEFINED

ANATOMY
The study of the body parts or structures

PHYSIOLOGY
The study of how the structures work

The body is composed of cells which in turn form tissue, which in turn forms structures/organs, that form systems, that form humans.

1.   THE SKELETAL SYSTEM
The framework or scaffolding of the body is the skeletal system. Composed of bones, ligaments (ligaments join bone to bone), and joints (where bones meet).

Main function
Assists locomotion, protects internal structures, acts as a reservoir for minerals and produces blood cells.

2.   THE MUSCULAR SYSTEM
The clothing or meat of the body is the muscular system. As its name suggests it is composed of the muscles of the body plus the tendons which are extensions of the muscle and which join muscle to bone.

Main function
Aids locomotion, maintains posture, gives shape to the body and protects internal structures.

3.   THE NERVOUS SYSTEM
Formed by the brain, spinal cord (central nervous system) and the peripheral nervous system.

Function - often likened to an office telephone system, the nervous system carries messages and commands throughout the body. It is the most complex of all systems and as a result probably the least understood.

4. THE LIQUID SYSTEM
The Vascular or Circulatory system and the Lymphatic system.

Cardio Vascular System
Formed by blood, blood vessels and the heart.

Function - to maintain life through the circulation of nutrients and oxygen and the removal of waste.

Lymphatic system
Formed by lymph vessels (similar to blood vessels), lymph tissue and lymph nodes.

Function - to assist in waste removal and fighting infection.

5 RESPIRATORY SYSTEM (BREATHING SYSTEM)
Formed by the lungs and airways including those of the mouth and nose.

Main Function
To maintain life by the inhalation of oxygenated air for circulation by the blood, and the exhalation of carbon dioxide given up by the blood.

6 DIGESTIVE SYSTEM (THE FOOD MACHINE)
Formed by the mouth, oesophagus, stomach, small intestine, large intestine (bowel), liver, gall bladder and pancreas.

Main function
To take in and process food, absorb nutrients and excrete the waste.

7   URINARY SYSTEM
   (FLUID DISPOSAL)

Formed by the Kidneys, Ureter tubes, Bladder and Urethra.

Main Function
To extract waste products from the blood and excrete them and to maintain the composition and volume of blood.

8   GENITO SYSTEM (REPRODUCTIVE)
   (THE GENE MACHINE)

Formed by the male and female reproductive glands.
Female Ovaries and Uterus
Male Testes, Penis, Prostrate and Vas Deferens

9   ENDOCRINE SYSTEM (THE HORMONE OR CHEMICAL SYSTEM)

Formed by a group of glands each with a specific function to secrete hormones/chemicals directly into the blood stream to reach a particular target organ. i.e. :

Hypothalamus	Adrenals
Pituitary	Ovaries / Testes
Parathyroid	Pancreas / Islets of Langerhans
Thyroid	

THE SKIN - NOT A SYSTEM

The overcoat or wrapping is the skin. The skin protects the internal structures. It contains tactile nerve endings to make us aware of our environment, i.e. heat, cold, pressure, pain. The skin also contains appendages or extensions each with a valued function. Sweat glands help regulate the body's temperature; sebaceous or oil glands lubricate skin and hair; the hair follicle (tunnel) for hair growth and the exit channel for sebum. Facial and body hair helps to regulate body temperature and hair also has a protective role i.e. protects the head from the elements. Nails protect the tips of fingers and toes.

SOME HELPFUL DIAGRAMS

RIGHT FOOT
(Sole)

Shoulder
Arm
Knee
Hip
Lower Back

Spine

200

ZONES OF THE HAND

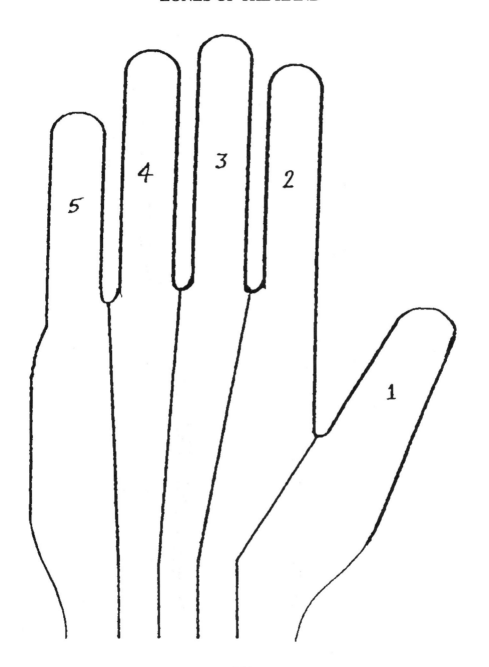

RIGHT HAND
(Back)

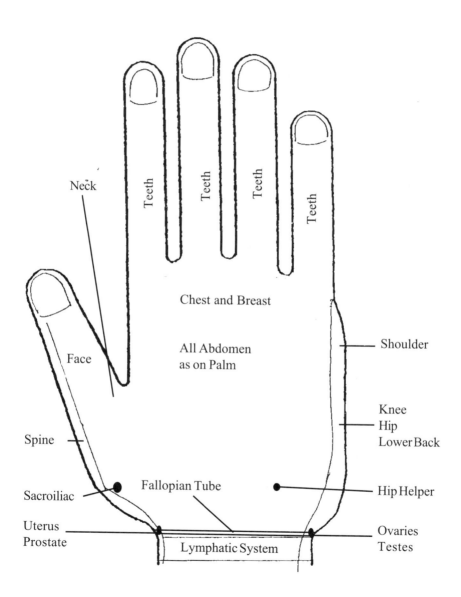

Neck

Teeth

Teeth

Teeth

Teeth

Chest and Breast

All Abdomen
as on Palm

Face

Shoulder

Spine

Knee
Hip
Lower Back

Sacroiliac

Fallopian Tube

Hip Helper

Uterus
Prostate

Ovaries
Testes

Lymphatic System

LEFT HAND
(Back)

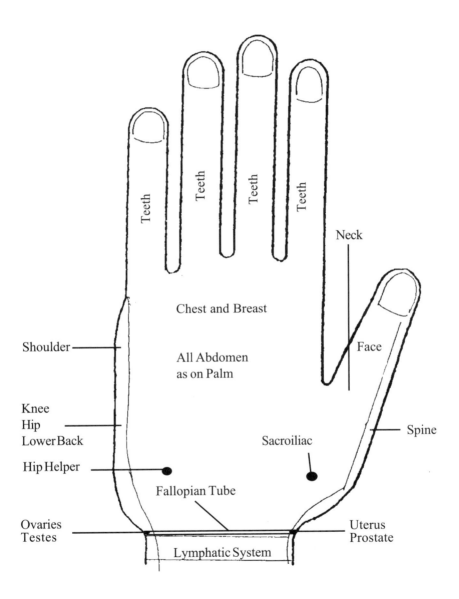

Teeth

Teeth

Teeth

Teeth

Neck

Chest and Breast

Shoulder

Face

All Abdomen
as on Palm

Knee
Hip
Lower Back

Spine

Sacroiliac

Hip Helper

Fallopian Tube

Ovaries
Testes

Uterus
Prostate

Lymphatic System

RIGHT HAND
(Palm)

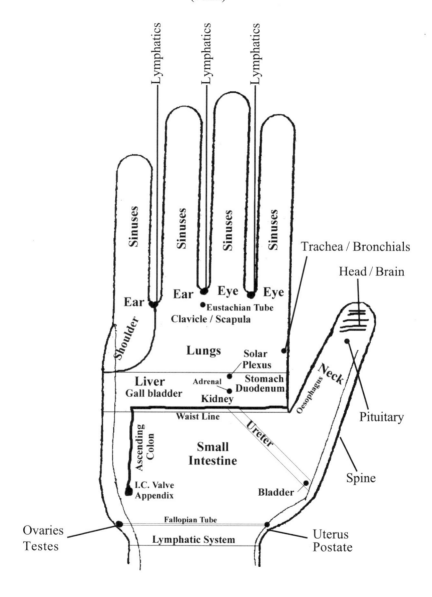

Lymphatics
Lymphatics
Lymphatics

Sinuses
Sinuses
Sinuses
Sinuses

Trachea / Bronchials

Head / Brain

Ear
Ear
Eye
Eye

• Eustachian Tube

Clavicle / Scapula

Shoulder

Lungs
Solar
Plexus

Liver
Adrenal
Stomach
Gall bladder
Duodenum
Kidney

Neck
Oesophagus

Waist Line

Ureter

Pituitary

Ascending
Colon

Small
Intestine

Spine

I.C. Valve
Appendix

Bladder

Ovaries
Testes

Fallopian Tube

Lymphatic System

Uterus
Postate

LEFT HAND
(Palm)

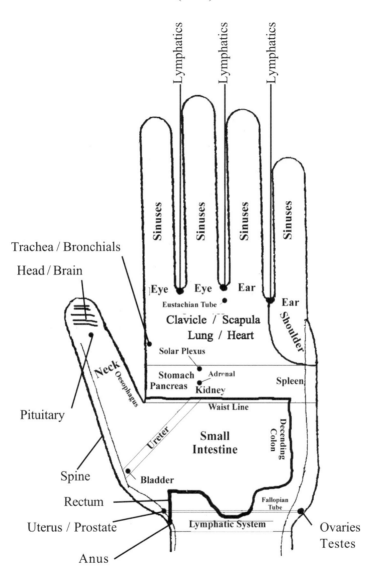

Lymphatics

Lymphatics

Lymphatics

Sinuses

Sinuses

Sinuses

Sinuses

Trachea / Bronchials

Head / Brain

Eye Eye Ear

Eustachian Tube

Ear

Shoulder

Clavicle / Scapula

Lung / Heart

Solar Plexus

Neck

Oesophagus

Stomach Adrenal

Pancreas

Kidney

Spleen

Pituitary

Waist Line

Ureter

Small
Intestine

Decending
Colon

Spine

Bladder

Rectum

Fallopian
Tube

Uterus / Prostate

Lymphatic System

Ovaries
Testes

Anus

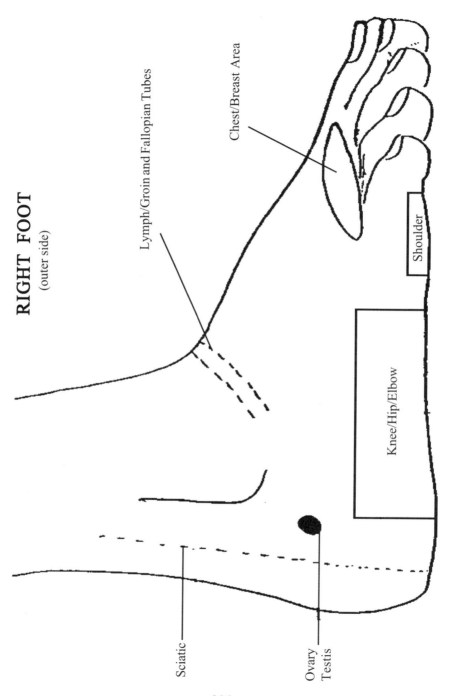

RIGHT FOOT
(outer side)

Chest/Breast Area

Lymph/Groin and Fallopian Tubes

Shoulder

Knee/Hip/Elbow

Sciatic

Ovary
Testis

206

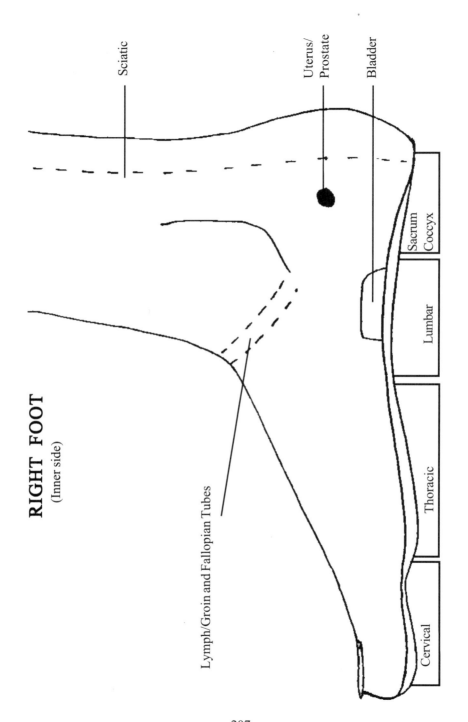

RIGHT FOOT
(Inner side)

Sciatic

Uterus/
Prostate

Bladder

Sacrum
Coccyx

Lumbar

Thoracic

Cervical

Lymph/Groin and Fallopian Tubes

207

SOME HOLDING TECHNIQUES

SOME HOLDING TECHNIQUES

BENDING BACK THE TOES

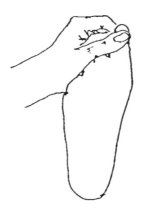

HOLDING TECHNIQUE WHEN TREATING
CHEST OR ABDOMEN

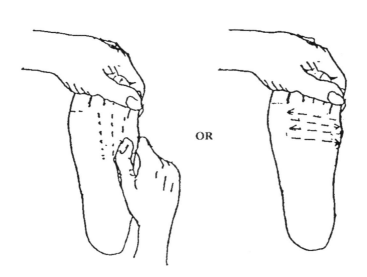

OR

FOOT SUPPORT / HOLDING TECHNIQUE

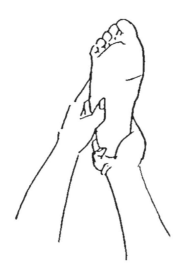

A HOLDING TECHNIQUE

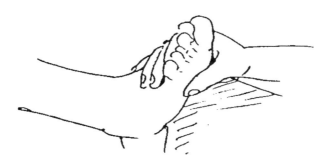

WORKING ON SOLAR PLEXUS

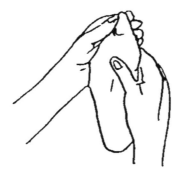

FINDING A SCHOOL OR A PROFESSIONALLY QUALIFIED REFLEXOLOGIST

The International Federation of Reflexologists (IFR) has been in existence since 1985 offering professional guidance, training courses and examinations. The examination to prove ability in both the theory and practice of Reflexology. For the IFR these professional examinations are now validated by the **International Examination Board.**

Anatomy & Physiology study is compulsory for all IFR students. The standard achieved in this subject is equivalent to A level. At the time of printing the IFR is the only Reflexology professional body that requires this level of training.

Further training that forms part of an accredited course includes basic clinical pathology, business management, first aid, an understanding of other complementary therapies and the ability to communicate with the orthodox medical profession.

If you would like to receive details of your (geographically) closest school or professionally qualified therapist then contact the IFR. The address and telephone number are listed at the back of this book.

GENERAL NOTES ON BECOMING A QUALIFIED REFLEXOLOGIST

As I have said before, it is not easy to learn Reflexology from a book.

For the Therapist who would like to work as a professional I would venture to say it is almost impossible without years of practise, trial and error to achieve the standard of a professional without some help and guidance in the practical and theoretical field.

No book which I have found, or indeed this one which I myself have written, can possibly contain all the information on reflexology reactions to treatments, anatomy, physiology, disorders and diseases.

A course of Reflexology for the professional Therapist will answer all these questions. It will also give the student time for practical and theoretical work whilst under supervision.

All budding Reflexologists with a thirst for knowledge who do not hold a qualification in anatomy and physiology should buy and study a simple textbook on the subject ; and it would be even more advantageous if the opportunity presents itself, to attend a part time course (day or evening) in Human Biology at your local college/school of Continuing Education and Training. Either or both of these courses of action will make life much easier when and if you decide to become a professional Therapist.

One other book which I feel sure would be invaluable is a good simple to follow Medical Dictionary.

Practising Reflexologists are required to hold a certificate in First Aid.

Recommended courses : Nutrition for the practitioner
                       Counselling skills for the practitioner

STUDENT NOTES

STUDENT NOTES

STUDENT NOTES

ADDRESSES OF ORGANISATIONS

(enclose A4 size s.a.e. with Enquiry)

The International Federation of Reflexologists
76 - 78 Edridge Road
Croydon
Surrey
England
CR0 1EF
Tel : 0181 667 9458

International Examination Board. (I.E.B.)
1 Northumberland Avenue
Trafalgar Square
London
WC2N 5BW
Tel : 0171 872 5456

Complementary therapies courses

Colette McCabe,
Rathganny
Multy Farnham,
Co. West Meath,
Ireland.

Renée Tanner
Principal
Renbardou Beauty and Complementary Therapies Training Centre.
Acorn House,
Cherry Orchard Road,
Croydon, Surrey, England CR0 6BA
Tel : 0181 686 4781

OTHER RELATED PUBLICATIONS BY RENÉE TANNER

BOOKS

Step by Step	Aromatherapy	By Renée Tanner
Step by Step	Basic Anatomy & Physiology for Students	By Renée Tanner
Step by Step	Basic Massage	By Renée Tanner
Reflexology	The Case History Book	By Renée Tanner

VIDEOS

Step by Step	Aromatherapy	By Renée Tanner
Step by Step	Reflexology	By Renée Tanner
Step by Step	Massage	By Renée Tanner
Step by Step	Facial Massage	By Renée Tanner

POSTERS

Foot Reflexology Chart	By Renée Tanner
Hand Reflexology Chart	By Renée Tanner

Available from :

Douglas Barry Publications
21 Laud Street
Croydon, Surrey. CR0 1SU
Tel : 0181 680 9631 Fax: 0181 681 3834